AGELESS
STRENGTH

AGELESS STRENGTH

STRONG AND FIT
FOR A **LIFETIME**

JEFF HOROWITZ

VELO.
press

Boulder, Colorado

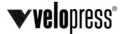

3002 Sterling Circle, Suite 100
Boulder, CO 80301–2338 USA

VeloPress is the leading publisher of books on endurance sports. Focused on cycling, triathlon, running, swimming, and nutrition/diet, VeloPress books help athletes achieve their goals of going faster and farther. Preview books and contact us at velopress.com.

Distributed in the United States and Canada by Ingram Publisher Services

A Cataloging-in-Publication record for this book is available from the Library of Congress.
ISBN 978-1-937715-71-7

This paper meets the requirements of ANSI/NISO Z39.48-1992 (Permanence of Paper).

Art direction and design: Vicki Hopewell
Photography: Jason Innes, cover and interior, except Rugile Kaladyte, p. 37; Brad Kaminski, p. 38;
    iStock, pp. viii, 25
Cover design: Kristin Weber
Composition: Jessica Xavier
Illustrations: Charlie Layton, pp. 34, 35

17   18   19 / 10   9   8   7   6   5   4   3   2   1

Strength for balance
Balance for health
Health for life

CONTENTS

INTRODUCTION: AGING BODIES, AGELESS STRENGTH 1

1 A NEW WAY OF UNDERSTANDING EXERCISE 10

2 CHANGES AND CHALLENGES 20

3 YOUR BODY, YOUR EQUIPMENT 30

4 THE PROGRAM 40

5 THE EXERCISES 46
   BALANCE STRENGTH FUNCTIONAL

6 THE WORKOUTS 156

7 STRENGTH FOR THE LONG TERM 188

Acknowledgments 197
Exercise Index 199
Notes 203
About the Author 206

THE EXERCISES

BALANCE 51

STRENGTH 89

FUNCTIONAL 135

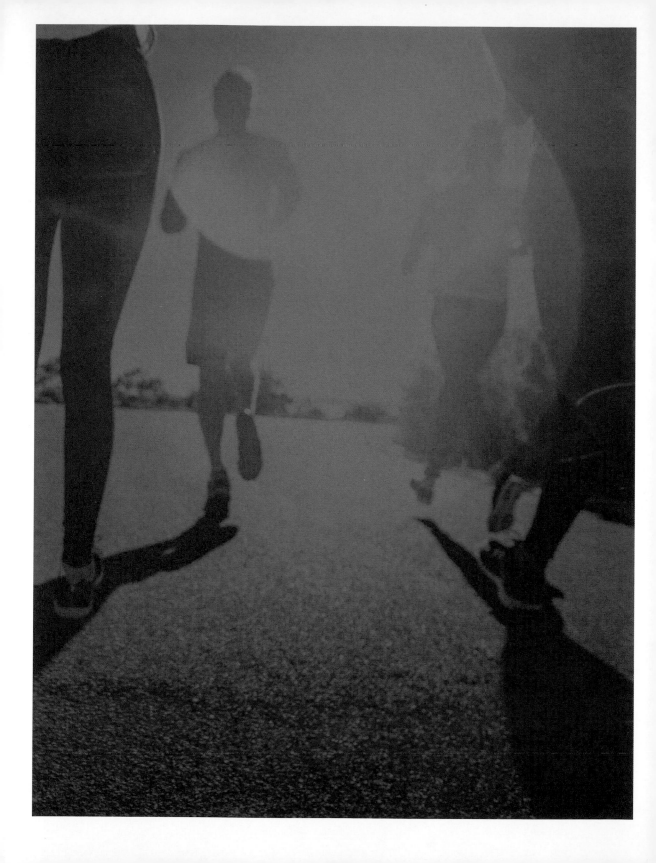

AGING BODIES, AGELESS STRENGTH

There's a common belief that once we cross over the great divide of 40, the years bring only greater physical decline as we journey toward the big dirt sleep. Vitality drains away year by year as we sit idly by, like crabs in a pot of water over a flame. As we become more and more reliant on canes, wheelchairs, and caretakers, we lose strength, independence, and quality of life.

This isn't a pleasant view of the golden years. I don't buy it, and neither should you.

Yes, physical changes come along with age. But we don't have to accept all of these changes as inevitable, and we certainly don't have to give the Grim Reaper a helping hand before our time. With a little focused effort, we can maintain vitality and strength throughout our advancing years, and in some cases achieve the best fitness of our lives.

To understand how this can be true, we need to understand how the body works and the difference between our potential fitness and our actual fitness.

The body functions on a "use it or lose it" basis: Without a challenge to fight against, the body wastes away. This process is called *atrophy*, and it's a natural law of conservation. What our bodies don't need, they lose. That includes muscle, bone, endurance, and fitness.

Luckily, it doesn't take a lot of work to keep our bodies working well. As we go about our daily routines, our bodies are being challenged in many ways, and they respond appropriately. Like a big city that never sleeps, the body is never truly at rest, despite appearances to the contrary. Every minute of every day, for example, our bodies fight off invading microbes. While we sleep, our bodies are in their highest repair mode, releasing human growth hormone to trigger the repair of damaged and injured tissue, and rebuild worn-out muscle and bone. If we had to monitor all of this activity consciously, we'd be overwhelmed, but our bodies handle these monumental tasks in stride.

At least they do when we're younger. As we get older, things begin to change. Our bodies begin to release less human growth hormone during our sleep,[1] and we need more time to recover from big workouts.

Discouraged? Don't be, because that's not the full story. Even with a diminished capacity to repair, the body can always change for the better. At *any* age, it can respond to physical stimuli—that is, exercise—by resculpting itself to handle a new challenge.

Consider this example: If a teenager and a 50-something both began a running program, each would probably feel a bit sore at first, but the older runner might need an extra day of rest every week. Yet after a month or two, they'd both find their earlier workouts to be much easier and would be ready for more challenging runs. During their weeks of training, both would experience a wide range of changes, whether they were aware of them or not. These would include an increase in blood volume to deliver more nutrients and oxygen to working muscles, an increase in the number of mitochondria in their muscle cells to deliver more energy to power contraction of muscle cells, and an increase in sweat rate so they could cool off more efficiently.

This is the essence of exercise: the gradual, measured overload of the body's capacity to do work, which triggers an adaptation response. Work a little harder, and your body will change itself to make your job easier.

Here's the important point: That process is not limited to the young. It can occur any time, for anyone.

Unfortunately, this works in the other direction as well. If we fail to do the minimal amount of work necessary to trigger maintenance of our fitness, we lose the capacity to do that work. That, too, is true at any time, for anyone.

This phenomenon is perhaps most dramatically demonstrated by astronauts living on the International Space Station.[2] Their bodies lose muscle mass and strength while they are in space since they no longer have to fight against the demands of gravity. These changes could compromise their long-term health and make their adjustment back to living on Earth difficult, so they spend hours of every 24-hour "day" tethered to fitness machines to keep as fit as they can.

For those of us stuck on Earth, the challenges are less dramatic but no less real. The demands of office jobs and the temptations of our virtual reality–based culture have made us increasingly sedentary, with the result that our bodies no longer feel pushed to maintain high levels of strength and fitness. This trend only accelerates as we enter middle age and beyond.

You might think that when faced with this situation, people would conclude that they need to become more active to restore health and vitality. But that's often not the case. Many people seem to believe that as they get older, they should be more careful about what they do and take even fewer chances with their bodies. Believing that exertion can bring strain and injury, they avoid challenging activities.

But as we now know, following this path leads to the exact opposite result. Instead of being safer and healthier by avoiding exercise, older people become less fit and more at risk for injury and disease. Their lifestyle then yields a self-fulfilling prophecy: They slow down because they think they should, given their age, and then their bodies lose fitness and slow down too.

Instead, they should ramp up their activity. They might need to be smarter about what they do—that's what this book is all about—but middle age shouldn't mark the end of challenging activity. It should instead mark the start of the next chapter. In fact, rather than being a time of declining fitness, our mature years can be a time for improvement.

EXERCISE AND MENTAL HEALTH

Exercise improves physical strength, functionality, and quality of life, but that's not all. Scientists have now determined conclusively that regular exercise is also one of the most effective tools to improve mental health.

Anyone who has ever engaged in a regular exercise routine can attest to the generally improved sense of well-being that exercise brings—a version of the "runner's high" that was first recognized during the running boom of the 1970s. Engaging in a regular exercise program often involves learning new skills and demonstrating commitment, which in turn raises self-esteem. Exercise has also been shown to improve sleep, reduce stress, and improve memory.

But the effects of exercise go beyond even those positive results. Studies have shown that exercise can help reduce the effects of clinical depression, anxiety, attention deficit hyperactive disorder, and post-traumatic stress disorder.

How is this possible? Because exercise not only promotes adaptive changes in our muscles and neural pathways, it also affects brain chemistry. Exercise increases the release of anti-inflammatory hormones and causes an increase in endorphins, those powerful chemicals that provide us with an emotional lift. Exercise also boosts the brain's levels of dopamine, norepinephrine, and serotonin, all of which have a profound effect on our ability to concentrate.

Behaviorally, exercise provides a powerful distraction from our usual thought patterns, which can allow us to break from negative habits and enable us to see new ways of looking at old problems. Exercise also helps us relax by releasing muscular stress.[3]

Whatever the reasons for our negative feelings—hormonal, psychological, or behavioral—for many people, the most satisfying moment of the day comes when they successfully complete a challenging workout. After all, so many elements of daily life are ambiguous. The security and pleasure of our relationships, our parenting, or our jobs can sometimes be unclear, but there is nothing ambiguous about doing 20 perfect repetitions of an exercise that only a month earlier we were unable to do. In moments like that, we feel a sense of accomplishment that could last all day. That's good medicine.

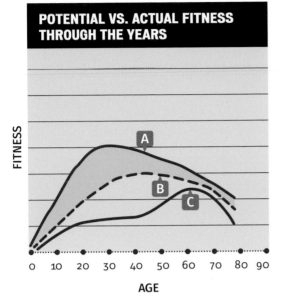

POTENTIAL VS. ACTUAL FITNESS THROUGH THE YEARS

FITNESS

A

B

C

0   10   20   30   40   50   60   70   80   90

AGE

Take a look at the chart, Potential Vs. Actual Fitness Through the Years. The vertical axis represents fitness, and the horizontal axis represents age. The higher the point on the chart, the greater the fitness, and the farther the point is to the right, the older the person is. A single point on this chart represents a person's fitness level at a particular point in time, and a connected series of dots—the arcs in this chart—represents a person's fitness during the course of his or her lifetime. In a chart like this, the person whose fitness is being measured has two arcs: one representing *potential* fitness and another representing *actual* fitness.

We'll define *potential fitness* as the theoretical upper limit of a person's strength and fitness. In the chart, the arc **A** represents our collective potential fitness. In reality, potential fitness varies from person to person, mirroring the differences in our physical gifts and life situations. But in general, the shape of this arc reflects potential fitness for nearly everyone.

As you can see, arc **A** peaks in our mid- to late twenties, and then it begins a steady decline, with a sharp drop-off late in life.[4] You might look at this curve and conclude that your physical peak was early in life and that you'll never be as strong and fit as you were back in your youth.

In all likelihood, you would be wrong. That's because most people don't come close to their potential fitness. This is particularly true earlier in life, when the temptations of junk food and alcohol, combined with a lack of knowledge about healthy choices, can leave many people well below their ideal fitness levels.

Now look at arc **B**. That curve represents a hypothetical person's actual fitness throughout his or her life.

The gap between **A** and **B** is shown by the blue shaded area, which represents our fitness gap. It marks the difference between where we actually are in life and where we could be if we worked to improve our health and fitness.

As luck would have it, arc **B** mirrors my own fitness history. I spent my high school and college years well above my ideal weight, with only a passing interest in regular exercise. As you can see, that left me well below my potential.

But then a curious thing happened. I discovered a love for running and exercise. I lost weight and got fit. As time went on, I learned more about what worked for me and what didn't. Even as I entered middle age, when I was supposedly past my peak potential fitness, my actual fitness was still on the rise.

For some people, late-life changes in their actual fitness can be even more dramatic. Look at arc **C**. Let's call the person represented by this arc Sarah. For many years, Sarah was stuck in an unhealthy lifestyle. Let's imagine that Sarah spent those years pursuing her career and raising a family. By necessity, Sarah put her health on the back burner, as many of us do, since there are only so many hours in a day and there is so much to be done.

But when Sarah turned 50, she resolved to get her health on track. She began exercising regularly and eating better. By the time she hit retirement age, she was actually healthier and more fit than she'd ever been, and feeling great.

Now what if Sarah had known about her potential fitness arc? Her feel-good story might have turned out very differently. She might have gotten discouraged and never started her program. Instead, she didn't think about how her potential fitness was lower at age 50 than at 25. And as a result, she began working out in middle age, and she changed her life.

The key fitness goal for each of us is to do what Sarah did: reduce the difference between our potential fitness arc and our actual fitness arc, at whatever age we find ourselves. However, just as perfection is a laudable but ultimately unattainable goal, so too is the goal of fully living up to our physical potential. This shouldn't stop us from aiming for it and raising ourselves up as high as we possibly can.

Whatever new level we achieve allows us to enjoy our lives to the greatest degree possible. Instead of spending our golden years complaining about aches and pains, we can spend them pursuing new adventures and challenges.

You might ask how this goal is different from a younger person's training goal. It isn't. Improving fitness is appropriate for everyone at every age.

In this sense, *Ageless Strength* is not a training guide strictly for older people. Relegating it to an older demographic assumes older people should train in a way that doesn't apply to younger people. That's simply not the case. However, our mature years bring more urgency to addressing specific challenges. We'll spend time discussing those later in the book.

Keep in mind that older versions of our bodies are not fundamentally different from younger versions. Our bodies work the same way now as they did then, and they respond the same way to exercise. Aging simply brings fewer margins for error. In our youth, we had the luxury of being able to be less mindful of our health and suffered few if any consequences for inattentiveness or poor decisions. As older adults, we need to be smarter about what we do and how we do it.

So would this book also work for younger athletes? Absolutely. I wish I had followed a program like this much earlier in my life. That leaves open the question of what each of us would have been like if we had followed this program when we were much younger, when we were at a point of higher potential.

A few people might know those dedicated, elite young athletes who have reduced their fitness gap to a sliver. But even those people might not enjoy overall health. In their pursuit of excellence, elite athletes often sacrifice key aspects of their overall fitness and then suffer the consequences. There are plenty of stories of young gymnasts, baseball players, and football players who have blown out their shoulders and knees and are already on prescription painkillers.

For the rest of us, playing the "what might have been" game is an interesting distraction, but it shouldn't consume us. Our focus is on being the best we can be going forward. If we don't assume any limits to our actual fitness now or in the future, we could end up being surprised at what we can achieve.

Let's get started.

CENTENARIAN MARATHONER
FAUJA SINGH

Fauja Singh was born on April 1, 1911, in Punjab, a region in pre-partition British India. He was the youngest of four children. He had thin, weak legs and did not walk until he was five years old, although he took up running for a time as a young man. The son of a rural farmer, he became a farmer himself, married, and fathered six children. Like so many of his neighbors and friends, Fauja never learned to read or write.

Fauja's wife died in 1992, but it was the death of one of his sons from a workplace accident in August 1994 that sent Fauja into a depression. At the urging of his family, he emigrated to England shortly afterward to live with another of his sons.

There, at 89 years of age, Fauja took up running again. After completing a race that he believed was 20 miles (it was probably only 20 kilometers), he decided to run a marathon. A practicing Sikh, Fauja was connected with a Sikh coach, Harmander Singh. When he showed up for his first training session, Fauja was dressed in a three-piece suit. Undeterred by Fauja's lack of knowledge even as to what kind of gear to wear, Harmander began the process of turning Fauja into a true runner.

Fauja's marathon debut was in the London Marathon in 2000. He completed it in 6 hours, 54 minutes. He ran the London Marathon again in 2001, 2002, and 2003. He achieved his best time in that race in 2003, at age 92, with a run of 6 hours, 2 minutes, setting a world record in his age group. Later that same year, he lowered the world record further when he completed the Toronto Waterfront Marathon in 5 hours, 40 minutes.

After these accomplishments, Fauja became a worldwide celebrity. In 2004 he was featured in an ad campaign by Adidas with the tagline "Impossible Is Nothing." He donated all of his earnings from his running career, including the Adidas sponsorship, to a children's charity.

And still Fauja ran. At age 100, at a special track meet set up in Toronto, Ontario, Canada, he set age-group world records at five distances in a 94-minute span: 200 meters (45.13), 400 meters (1:49.25), 800 meters (4:20.97), mile (9:40.13), and 3000 meters (18:38.48). He also ran the 100 meters (19.97), 1500 meters (11:27.81), and 5000 meters (31:31.12).

To put these accomplishments in perspective, consider his half-marathon personal best of 2 hours, 29 minutes, 59 seconds, which he posted in the 2004 Toronto Waterfront Half-Marathon. According to an age grade calculator, which uses effort-based formulas to compare times of older runners to those of runners in their prime, Fauja's effort was equivalent to a young elite runner posting a half-marathon time of 45:59. The current world record for the half-marathon is 58:23, set in 2010. Fauja's projected time would be at a pace of 3:30.37 per mile. In contrast, the world record in the mile currently stands at 3:43.13.

But Fauja wasn't yet done. His trainer had him cut back on his racing in order to save up for a historic effort. On October 16, 2011, Fauja ran the Toronto Waterfront Marathon in 8:11:06, becoming the first 100-year-old to finish a marathon. The following summer he was selected for the honor of participating in the Olympic torch relay.

The closer you look at Fauja's accomplishments, the more amazing they are revealed to be. Yet despite these accomplishments, Fauja is not an imposing man physically or temperamentally. He is average height, five foot eight, but is very slight, weighing only 115 pounds. He neither smokes nor drinks alcohol, and he follows a simple vegetarian diet. His routine consists of running on weekends, taking long walks during the week, and doing some calisthenics regularly.

Not surprisingly, Fauja has encountered many people along the way who thought that an elderly man shouldn't engage in long-distance running. "I decided to ignore them on the advice of my coach, as it stopped me responding to what I considered to be negativity," he said. "I did, however, remind people that while I was getting fitter and stronger, they were deteriorating, and we all were going to die someday anyway."

As of this writing, Fauja, aged 106, has retired from racing. But he has not stopped running. His accomplishments—all achieved after he was in his ninth decade—are proof of the human body's ability to respond to exercise and improve at any age.

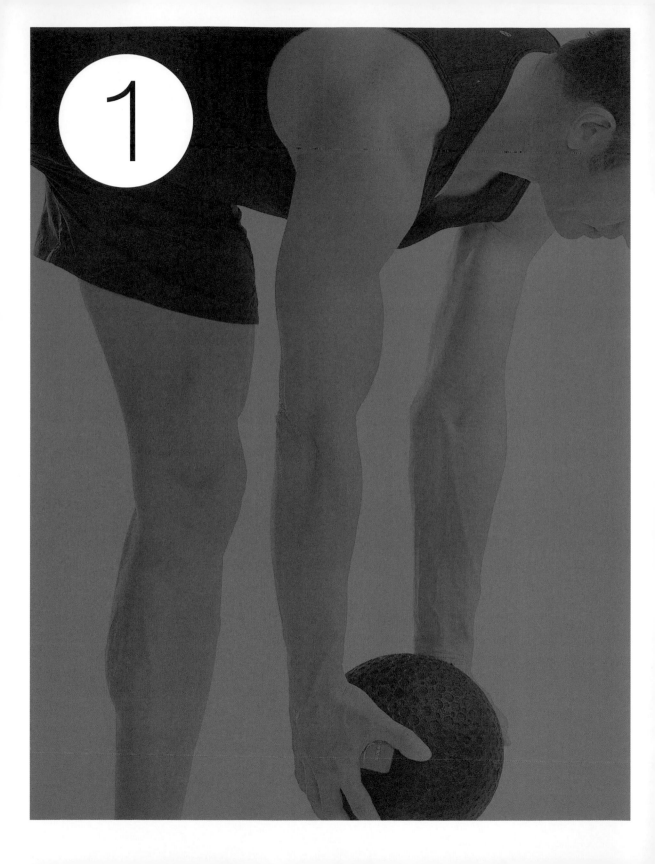

A NEW WAY OF
UNDERSTANDING EXERCISE

If you are looking to build massive arm, back, and chest muscles, you're in the wrong place. That's bodybuilding, and plenty of good books out there explain how to train for that. Our goal here is different.

This book aims not to help you build a bulging body but rather to build health and fitness for the long term, the kind of sustainable fitness that will enable you to enjoy life for decades to come. To do that, we're going to have to forget everything we thought we knew about exercise and look at workouts in a completely new way.

MEET YOUR BRAIN

In the traditional mode of strength training, you aim to isolate particular muscles and repeatedly put them through a range of motion, working against resistance, often using a dumbbell or a barbell. The movements are generally simple—an arm curl or a bench press—and they are performed to failure, which is the point at which a person is no longer able to perform that particular movement at that particular resistance level.

There's nothing wrong with this approach. Every day, thousands of people work out in this mode, and many of them get good results. But we can do better. To understand how, let's take this step by step.

First, imagine that you and your body aren't a single unit but instead are separate people occupying the same space, like college roommates. It's not really that strange an idea. After all, your body already handles many functions and solves many problems without asking for your conscious permission or input. For example, your body jacks up your heart rate when you climb stairs, gives you an adrenaline surge when you're scared, and cools you off with sweat when you're hot.

Similarly, if you were in a potentially life-threatening crisis, your body would decide what drastic measure to take to preserve your life, such as cutting blood flow to your hands and feet in order to reduce loss of core body heat if you were freezing, even though this puts your fingers and toes at risk of frostbite. To your body, that's a fair trade.

The act of drowning presents an even starker example. After initial immersion in water, a victim may panic and gasp for air. If he swallows some water, he will cough it up and try to keep his mouth closed. After a very short time, however, the buildup of carbon dioxide will trigger a breathing reflex. In other words, the victim's body will decide that the risk of keeping its mouth closed is greater than the risk of opening it. This makes sense, since the lack of air from keeping the mouth closed will certainly cause death, while opening the mouth may not.

After involuntarily opening his mouth, the drowning victim will find water instead of air. When that water is inhaled and reaches the lower part of the airway, it will trigger a throat spasm. That's the body's way of protecting the lungs. With the pathway to the lungs sealed off, the water will instead be routed to the stomach. This could make the drowning victim sick, but it will buy him a few more moments to find air.

But if there's no air to be had, the crisis will deepen. The victim will lose consciousness. His throat will then relax, allowing water to fill his lungs. At this point, the body will begin to shut down its organs one by one, saving the brain—its most important organ—for last. Every moment now brings more irreversible damage. Eventually, there's nothing more the body can do to preserve the victim's life. But it will have done its best, following a rational plan about which the victim was completely unaware.

If these examples seem dramatic to you, that's because to the body, all of life is a struggle for survival. The body doesn't understand the idea of play and exercise. It assumes that everything you do is linked to your effort to either get food or to avoid being food. Your body's goal is to navigate these challenges and do all that it can to help preserve your life.

With this in mind, let's take a trip to a local gym and look around. We see a lot of people working out: Over there is a guy working on his arms by doing biceps curls with a barbell, and back there is a woman doing a dumbbell chest press. Over there is a man doing pull-ups. It's all very impressive, until we look closer and see that all three of these people are using poor form.

The guy working his arms is swinging his body and leaning back as he struggles to curl the barbell. The woman is arching her back and lifting her hips off the bench as she pushes against the dumbbells. The guy doing pull-ups is curling his body and swinging as he tries to rise up to the bar.

We know that all of this is wrong, but we know this as well: If we were to ask them *why* they are doing these very specific things—swinging the barbell, raising the hips up off the bench, curling and swinging the body—they would most likely be unable to tell us. They might not even be aware that they're cheating. So why are they doing these things?

Through this lens of our body-as-roommate, we can begin to answer these questions. The body assumes all of these movements—the curls, the chest presses, and the pull-ups—are related to survival, because why on earth would you be working so hard otherwise? To her body, then, the woman might be trying to push a boulder off her torso. To his body, the man doing pull-ups might be trying to find safety and shelter in a tree. Your body doesn't share the athlete's goal of isolating and improving individual muscles through resistance training. It is interested only in getting the work at hand done.

The body, in its wisdom, knows that there are three basic ways that it can achieve hard work quickly and easily:

- Involve as many muscle groups as possible
- Create momentum
- Seek out a mechanical advantage to increase leverage

To the body, all of this makes perfect sense. Involving more muscle groups makes it possible to generate more power without relying on any one muscle or muscle group to do all the work and risk strain or injury. Generating momentum encourages movement without using much energy, since the momentum carries the weight. And any mechanical advantage reduces the difficulty of moving the weight.

Let's look again at our three hapless athletes. We now can see that the guy doing curls is swinging his body because that will generate momentum to keep the barbell moving once he gets it started. He leans backward when the barbell is raised in order to let gravity pull it those final few inches toward his body. The woman doing chest presses, meanwhile, is raising her hips to change the angle of the exercise, which will help her engage additional muscles. If she does the repetitions quickly, she'll also get a rebound

effect at the bottom of the movement, giving her a few free inches of lift before she has to start working hard again. And the man doing pull-ups is curling his body to engage his abdominal muscles to help out his hardworking back. When he adds swinging to his movement, he's also generating momentum to carry his body up to the bar.

To the body, all of this makes sense, but for an athlete, these choices by the body raise the risk of injury because they create situations in which the body is moving faster than it should in a way that perhaps it should not, using muscles that might not be appropriate for the type of resistance that's been chosen. The body is willing to risk injury, though, because it believes that the athlete is doing something that absolutely needs to be done to preserve life, like eventually opening your mouth when you're under water for too long.

Many coaches and trainers address this problem by teaching their athletes how to use proper form by, for example, avoiding swinging their bodies or putting their bodies in risky positions. That makes perfect sense, but it's also throwing the baby out with the bathwater. Rather than ignore our body's wisdom, we can work *with* it to exercise in a manner that makes sense to our bodies and at the same time creates better, more sustainable fitness. To do so, we're going to rely on these principles in our workouts:

- Engage as many muscle groups as possible simultaneously
- Use momentum carefully to challenge muscles appropriately
- Reduce leverage and stability to encourage the body to work harder

By using these principles, we'll present the body with a way of exercising that will make more sense to it. One result will be that these movements will feel more natural. More important for long-term health and fitness, these movements will encourage the body to learn how to use its parts together in a way that is safe and builds appropriate strength.

This last point is subtle but important. When I was in high school, I lifted weights with my friends, as most boys in my neighborhood did. We did the traditional exercises, and we all got stronger and bigger, to a greater or lesser degree. Despite these improvements, however,

I never felt especially healthy. I did not become more athletic, did not move more gracefully, and did not become less clumsy. I was just a stronger version of the same old me.

Flash forward into the 21st century. I'm now a very different version of me. I am not as strong as I was then, at least as measured by the amount of weight that I can move with a bench press or squat. However, I've now got a body that performs very well in a very different way than it used to. I move with much more fluidity and control, and I can balance myself more easily. I'm not ashamed to take yoga classes anymore, and when I do, I don't make a fool of myself.

If I had to sum up the difference between the kind of body I had back then and the body I have now, I would say that before, my body felt like a collection of parts, but now it feels *integrated*. My brain has become the conductor of an orchestra, coordinating a roomful of musicians to create a wondrous symphony.

Well, maybe not a symphony. I'm not that good yet. But certainly a pleasing sound instead of a cacophony.

We've reached the point of our discussion when we can see the forest as distinct from the trees. What many people call "athletic grace" is no more than having a brain that is able to coordinate the body's movement—what exercise scientists call its *kinesthetic sense*, which is the brain's awareness of where the body is in space and in relation to gravity, and the brain's ability to use this information to balance and control the body in space.

The autonomous part of your brain that accomplishes this task—which I generally refer to simply as your body—uses muscles that are strong and familiar with the complicated task at hand. This athletic grace allows for very complex movements in sport, such as hitting a home run, nailing a jump shot, or winning a swim meet. But it's also used in everyday life when we move a piece of furniture, pick up a child, or paint a wall.

This kind of fitness is not for impressing people in the gym or for executing abstract movements like a bench press, which has little resemblance to the way in which we move in our everyday lives. It's for building the kind of body that can enjoy life outside the gym and stay as healthy and vibrant as possible for as long as possible.

Now let's talk about how we can get there.

LESS EXERCISE, MORE PROBLEM SOLVING

We now understand how the body behaves. Our next challenge is to figure out how to use the body in a way that makes sense to it but is also safe. To do this, we're going to have to stop thinking of exercise as just a series of sets and repetitions, and begin to think of it as a process of engaging the body and mind to problem solve. This involves understanding the three basic enablers of movement: the brain, the neural network, and the skeletal muscles.

To begin, let's review your personal history, from the beginning: You were born, and your brand-new little body came hardwired with a vast neural network connecting your brain to your muscles via a dense web of neurons. You were like a massive city with thousands of miles of roads. But at birth, the vast majority of these roads had not yet been traveled. The neural connection that would move your finger to your ear, for example, was not yet activated. You couldn't scratch an itch there even if you wanted to. You were a bundle of huge potential with very little ability.

For your parents, though, this was an amazing time. They got to see you explore your body and your environment, and slowly learn how to use this incredible machine that you were born with. You learned to roll over, crawl, and cruise along the wall.

After a few years, your neural network became increasingly activated. Your brain figured out the general layout of the city that is your body. It learned how to use the major highways to do things like walking and running, and it figured out how to use the avenues, streets, and alleyways to accomplish a wide range of other tasks, from feeding yourself to expressing emotion with your face.

As time passed, you began to specialize more and more, traveling over specific roadways more often while ignoring other roads completely. You learned to play the violin, perhaps, or dunk a basketball, or perform a plié. The result was that the most well-traveled roads became increasingly familiar while the ones that were less traveled, or ignored altogether, withered.

The science behind this process is understood fairly well. Neurons are the basic building blocks of the brain, and commands sent from these neurons to the different skeletal muscle cells of the body are carried along structures called axons,

which act as information highways. In their raw state, electrical impulses move openly along axons, losing energy as they go. But with repeated activation, axons develop a covering made of protein and fat called a myelin sheath. This sheath provides insulation, helping to maintain the strength and speed of the signal as it crosses over the axon. The more the neural network is engaged through repetition, the denser the sheath becomes. The result is a signal that retains its strength as it moves from your brain to your muscle, allowing the signal to stay clear, which prompts an increasingly more energetic and confident response from the muscle.

To understand this, think about the wires that connect speakers to receivers in an audio system. In a simple home system (at least in the old days), a basic thin wire would transmit the electrical impulse, which represented the music you had selected, from your receiver to your speakers. Better, more expensive cables would deliver a stronger signal, which would make the most of your stereo system's capability. These better cables were thicker, with thicker insulation covering them.

Your brain works in the same way, except that to improve the signal, it doesn't need to switch to new, better cables. It can simply improve the ones that it has.

This will be the key goal of much of our training: not only to improve strength but also to improve the ways in which we move. Our goal will be not just to get better at doing certain hard exercises and movements. We will also aim to master new movements, to go down those little-used streets and alleys in our neural city, so to speak. This will allow us to use the body in an increasingly wide range of ways, but without courting injury.

The ultimate goal of our workouts, then, to borrow the words of a coach whose name I've forgotten but whose wisdom I've long remembered, is to *expand our library of kinesthetic sense.*

Think on that for a moment. That's a wonderful image. Your body retains its familiarity with different movements much like a book collector keeps volumes in his library. Remember the old maxim that once you learn how to ride a bike, you never forget? To a large degree, it's true.

The more volumes you have in your kinesthetic library—meaning, the more movements that your body is familiar with—the greater your ability to move safely and gracefully in sport, work, and life. Every time we add a movement or a new wrinkle to an old movement, we expand this library, preparing ourselves to use our bodies in new ways if called upon to do so.

Here's an example. Last summer I spent a month in coastal Maine with my family. I used the time to run, hike, bicycle, and kayak, enjoying what my wife called Jeff-Camp. The kayaking was the most fun for me, because I love the feeling of exertion while I'm also enjoying the beautiful rocky shoreline. At one point, I needed to turn the kayak quickly, but instead of simply back paddling, I decided to try quickly rotating my hips, imitating a movement I often do on a machine I use in the gym back home. To my delight, the kayak flew around. All those repetitions I had performed at the gym had translated into a movement that was easily accessible to my brain's neural network when I decided that I needed to use it.

Here's another example: A few winters ago, my hometown of Washington, D.C., was hit by a snowstorm. When it blew over, I layered up and stepped outside to begin shoveling. As I lifted each shovelful of snow and twisted to dump it to the side, I felt more and more energized. I realized that this movement mimicked an exercise that I do with a dumbbell. My body knew exactly how to do this movement efficiently and with great power, and though I won't say that shoveling was as much fun as drinking hot chocolate afterward, it was much less of a chore than I thought it would be.

These are examples of functional strength, which I define as strength developed not for its own sake or for the performance of particular exercises, but in support of real-life activities. Whether you are kayaking or shoveling snow, moving furniture or trekking the Himalayas, this is the kind of strength that will make a difference to your quality of life in the long term.

Now here's the really interesting part: While much of the neural development that leads to specialization occurs early in life, scientists have discovered that this process can occur anytime, even in elderly adults.[1] If practice really does make perfect, as the science suggests, then some level of perfection can be achieved at any age. In other words, there is always the possibility that we can improve ourselves. The only thing stopping us is a reluctance to push out of our comfort zones.

Working toward improvement is not only desirable, it's something that our bodies actually crave. That's clear from the positive ways in which they respond to being pushed. If our bodies could talk, they might quote Shakespeare and say, "Now bid me run, and I will strive with things impossible. Yea, get the better of them."

Before we can ask our bodies to run, so to speak, we need to know in what direction we want them to move. In the next chapter we'll discuss the specific challenges that our bodies increasingly face with age. Once we understand these challenges, we can identify the exercises that we need to do to overcome them.

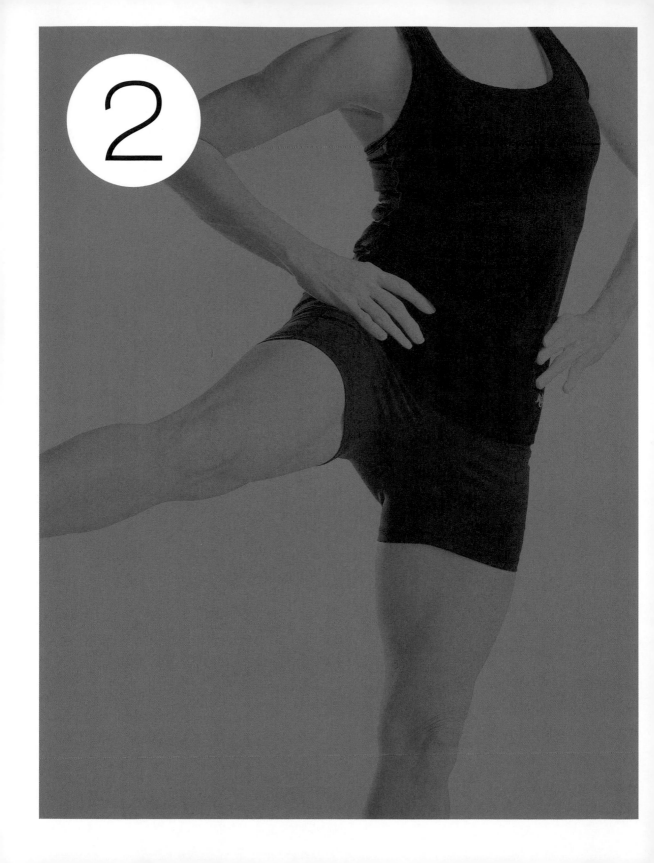

CHANGES
AND CHALLENGES

In the previous chapter we learned that our bodies work the same way when we're older as they do when we're younger. That's not to say that there are no differences at all. In many ways, our bodies may seem the same. Our organs, for example, still function the same way that they did when we were younger. But within this apparent sameness, our bodies do experience change. Skin loses elasticity, and hair loses pigment and begins to thin. And while these kinds of changes can be damaging to the ego, they do not threaten our health.

The same can't be said of other, less obvious changes that we experience to our muscle mass and strength, our bone health, and our balance. Changes in these three areas can impact our health. But the onset of change need not be feared, because we have ways to battle it every step of the way. For this reason, we won't call these changes threats, which implies potential helplessness. Instead, we'll call them challenges, because we possess the ability to meet these problems head on and deal with them. But first, we'll need to understand exactly what these challenges are.

MUSCLE MASS AND STRENGTH

As we saw in the potential versus actual fitness chart, potential fitness typically peaks during our mid- to late 20s. This is also the time when muscle mass, strength, and functionality generally peak as well, because up to that point our bodies are programmed to release hormones that cause continual growth of muscle.

As we enter our 30s, however, our bodies exit this programmed growth phase and we begin to run the risk of losing muscle mass and strength in a process called sarcopenia. From that point onward, we can lose as much as 3 to 8 percent of our muscle mass—or up to seven pounds of muscle—every decade.[1] That is, unless we do something to prevent that loss.

Many people aren't even aware that this loss is happening. That's because we need only a small fraction of our actual strength, 30 percent or so, to get through a typical day. Unless you've been doing something much more taxing, such as lifting weights, playing a sport at the elite level, or working in a very strenuous job, a 5 percent loss of strength wouldn't be immediately obvious because you'd still be able to easily climb stairs, wash your car, or move a box of clothes. But once this loss gets to 50 percent, the effects become much more apparent. Suddenly, tasks that once seemed easy, such as getting up from a couch, feel much harder.

Once this degeneration process begins, it only gets worse if left unchecked. The natural tendency at that point might be to avoid doing those things that feel difficult. But responding with a decrease in physical activity will only lead to further loss of muscle and a corresponding decrease in physical energy and stamina, as our aerobic capacity diminishes along with our strength. To this, add a tendency to gain weight and an overall decrease in health.

The effect of strength on overall health might not be immediately obvious. Muscle mass burns calories, so a decline in muscle tissue will cause a decrease in metabolic activity. This means that the body will burn fewer calories, which can affect insulin sensitivity and hormone levels. This in turn can lead to obesity, diabetes, and cardiovascular disease.

By our 60s and 70s, this loss of muscle mass and strength will have led to increased frailty and risk of falling, as well as decreased independence.

Inevitable? Happily, no. While we can't stop the age clock, we absolutely can change the way in which we age. Since muscle tissue can be regenerated at any age, we can use strength training to slow down the effects of aging and in some cases, even reverse them.[2] All it takes is a commitment to train just two to three times per week.[3] Make that commitment now, and we'll discuss the details of your workouts later in this book.

BONE DENSITY

The 206 bones that make up our skeletons provide structure, protection, and support for our bodies, and make movement possible. Despite appearing solid, however, our bones are actually a matrix of protein and minerals, comprised of living tissue that is constantly changing in a process known as remodeling. Specialized cells called osteoclasts break down older bone for reabsorption while other cells called osteoblasts bring protein and minerals—mostly calcium and phosphate—into the bone matrix for sculpting and repair.

During the arc of our lives, much of the cartilage that we're born with hardens into bone, small bones fuse, and all bones enlarge as we grow into adulthood. Nutrition and lifestyle, among other factors, help determine bone volume and density.

As with all living tissue, bone is susceptible to disease, as well as to disorders linked to insufficient density. One common ailment is osteoporosis, which is a reduction in bone mineral density that raises the risk of fracture. Postmenopausal women in particular are at risk for this disease, although it can strike men and premenopausal women as well.

Aging brings other challenges as well. Lubricating fluid in the joints may decrease, and cartilage may lose water content and become more susceptible to stress, especially in the hips and knees. This can lead to joint stiffness, loss of flexibility, and inflammation and arthritis. Vertebrae may compress, compromising posture and further limiting mobility. Over time, these changes can trigger a downward spiral in health.

But, once again, strength training can come to the rescue by reducing, delaying, and sometimes even reversing these outcomes. This is because strength training can add density and mineral content to aging bone.[4] It performs these miracles in a very straightforward way: by stressing

NUTRITION

Maintaining muscle mass and bone density is not just a matter of staying active; it also requires that you give your body the right raw materials for it to do its job once you've given it a training stimulus. That means eating the right foods.

Detailed nutritional recommendations are beyond the scope of this book, but we can discuss certain basic information to point you in the right direction. Current research indicates that some level of increased protein intake could help reduce the loss of muscle mass and would not pose any risk to our kidneys. However, it's unclear exactly how much additional protein we should eat.[5] Similarly, increased ingestion of calcium and related minerals such as magnesium could help delay, prevent, and reverse the onset of age-related bone density loss and osteoporosis.[6]

There's a lot of information available online and in books concerning nutrition, and much of it is contradictory. As a general rule, I tend to adopt the recommendations that have been accepted most widely by experts, and to view with skepticism any claims that promise quick and sudden results. As the old adage goes, if something sounds too good to be true, it probably is.

Our goal, then, should be to adopt an eating program that is sustainable and promises overall health, even if it doesn't deliver quick changes. Remember: Quick improvements can be followed by quick regressions, so any program that promises quick weight loss or gains is unlikely to help you maintain your improvements. The body responds best to incremental changes made over time. If you tend toward impatience, this might be hard to accept, but the gains you make will be gains that you'll be able to keep.

With this in mind, I'll offer a list of guidelines that will set you on the path to healthful eating:

- **Eat fresh.** Follow a diet that is low in processed foods and rich in variety. Fresh is better than packaged because no chemicals or preservatives are used in fresh food, and vitamins and nutrients tend to degrade over time, leaving older food less potent.
- **Don't rely on supplements.** Fresh food contains many beneficial compounds that can contribute to

our overall health; eating a vegetable containing vitamin C is better than taking a vitamin C pill.

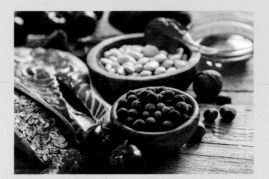

- **Eat breakfast.** Yes, our mothers were right. Breakfast is widely considered the most important meal of the day, and there is a strong coincidental link between eating breakfast and maintaining an appropriate body weight.
- **Keep the carbs.** About two-thirds of your food intake should consist of carbohydrates. This is the fuel that will power your workout, so don't skimp.
- **Remember protein.** Aim to eat half a gram to a full gram of protein for every pound of body weight. Protein is necessary for tissue repair and muscle growth, and it is essential for a healthy immune function. You don't need to be a slave to this formula; try to eat some quality protein with every meal.
- **Avoid sugar when possible.** There is little to no nutritional value in this simple carbohydrate, and although endurance athletes often rely on sugar for quick energy, it has no useful purpose in our daily lives. Ingesting sugar creates insulin spikes, which lowers insulin sensitivity in the body and raises the risk of diabetes.
- **Snack.** This is where out mothers were wrong. Eating healthy foods between meals keeps our blood sugar in balance and helps us control our appetites. Examples of healthy snacks include nuts, fruit, and whole-grain crackers.
- **Be mindful of fat.** There's a growing consensus that fat might have gotten a bad rap and that it's not the bogeyman that we've been led to believe it is. Indeed, some fat is absolutely essential for good health, and it can help provide us with a feeling of fullness. But keep in mind that fat is twice as calorie-dense as carbohydrates and protein are, so don't overdo your intake of this essential nutrient.

For more detailed recommendations, talk with your doctor or consult a licensed nutritionist.

the body and relying on the body's adaptive response. Just as with muscle, bones respond to resistance by getting tougher and stronger.

BALANCE

A friend of mine has a toddler whose given name is Cormac, but that's not what they call him. For now, at least, he goes by the name Tippy. He earned that because of the wobbly way that he teeters around the house and the consistency with which he lands on his bottom. That nickname will soon be outdated, though, as he finds his sea legs and learns how to negotiate his way through the world without any problems.

When Cormac is able to talk, he can thank three things for his mastery of balance: his vestibular system, his proprioceptive system, and his sight.

The *vestibular system* is based in Tippy's inner ear. It's a complex structure made up of chambers and tubes filled with fluid. Specialized nerves inside these structures gather information about the position of the body in relation to the pull of gravity.

The *proprioceptive system* uses nerve receptors in Tippy's skeletal muscles to gather information about the position of his body in space—everything from where his arms are to the position of his hips and the tilt of his head.

Finally, Tippy's *sight* also contributes to his balance. His depth perception, night vision, and sense of contrast will all be used by his brain, in conjunction with information from his vestibular system, to create a map of his surroundings in relation to his body's position.

Tippy's brain will process all of this data nearly instantaneously to determine the position of his body, and then it will use its neural network to engage the muscles that he needs to maintain his balance. As he moves, his brain will use the ongoing real-time data feed to constantly update his muscle contractions in order to maintain his balance. And voila! He's Tippy no more.

It's an amazing system, a true marvel of evolution. The precise way in which Tippy's brain will use his muscles to maintain balance is no less impressive.

The muscles that Tippy will primarily engage—which we all use daily—are his core muscles. These are found in his trunk, from mid-thigh to rib cage, on his front, back, and sides. They include hips, abdominals, and backside muscles.

Regarding balance, though, the undisputed champion of all these is the transverse abdominis.

The transverse abdominis is the deepest layer of muscle tissue in our midsection. It wraps around our bodies like a girdle. Whenever we move, the transverse abdominis clenches, holding our bodies in place as we move our arms and legs. It provides the anchor for our movement, giving us leverage to move without falling over.

Let's get interactive for a moment. Stand up and place a hand lightly on your stomach. While holding your hand very still, slowly draw in your stomach. Stop at the point when your hand is no longer in contact with your stomach. Maintain that position with your stomach and drop your hand. This contraction should be comfortable; there's no need to clench to the point of cramping.

You have activated your transverse abdominis. Remember this feeling. Once you gain the ability to activate this muscle on demand, you'll have a much easier time maintaining your balance during your workouts and, more importantly, in your daily life.

Tippy will be using his core muscles to maintain his balance for many decades to come. Eventually, though, his unsteadiness will return, as it will for all of us. That's because loss of balance is one of the key challenges that we face as we age. This is caused by degeneration of each of these systems: our visual acuity, our strength and the ability to use our strength effectively to control the position of our bodies in space, and the function of our inner ear.

As we age, these systems start to become compromised. Our sight, the ability to focus and see things clearly, diminishes with age. So do depth perception, night vision, and sensitivity to contrast. Eye problems can also impair, blur, or distort vision. The loss of these visual faculties compromises balance. The number of nerve cells in the vestibular system and blood flow to the inner ear also decrease after about age 55.

The loss of muscle strength is perhaps the most problematic. Most at risk are the fast-twitch muscle fibers, which provide explosive strength on demand, instantly. We rely on these muscles for quick adjustments in balance. When they're diminished, we're unable to catch ourselves easily when we stumble. When we were younger, we were able to use the muscle we had to adequately keep our balance, even if we were generally out of shape, but as we get older and lose muscle mass, we no longer have that luxury. Combined with diminished reflexes and coordination, we're increasingly likely to fall.

According to the Centers for Disease Control and Prevention, one out of four people age 65 and older experience a significant fall each year. An estimated 2.8 million older Americans seek emergency care each year due to a fall, and 800,000 of them are hospitalized because of their injuries. In addition, 300,000 older people are hospitalized annually for hip fractures, and 95 percent of these injuries were caused by a fall.

Falls are also the main cause of traumatic brain injuries in older people. Apart from the human cost of falls, consider the economic toll: Treatment for falls among older people costs $31 billion annually, two-thirds of which pays for fall-related hospitalization.[7]

No matter how you look at it, we simply cannot afford this situation.

THE ROAD BACK

If you find these changes discouraging, remember what I said earlier: You are not powerless to stop them. Research has found that less than 10 percent of Americans participate in regular exercise, and the most sedentary group is older than 50. That's the problem. Research shows that much of what we thought was age-related deterioration is really the result of sedentary lifestyles and the development of medical conditions rather than of aging itself. The problems stem more from disuse than from simple aging.

This puts the control is back in our hands. Deterioration and its concomitant problems are not inevitable. When we exercise, at any age, we improve muscle tone, increase range of motion, improve posture, increase bone mass, increase coordination, decrease blood pressure, improve weight control, reduce the incidence of low-back pain, improve sleep patterns, and improve functional ability. Not surprisingly, these changes also bring greater independence and improved self-esteem.[8]

The studies on the beneficial effects of exercise have focused on older adults and have targeted those who exhibit signs of deterioration. But we don't have to wait until we develop significant problems before we act. The sooner we begin training for strength, the sooner we'll reap the benefits and delay the onset of deterioration.

AEROBIC CONDITIONING AND AGING

One of the other effects of aging is the loss of aerobic fitness. Over time, we lose cardiovascular capacity as our attainable maximal heart rate and stroke volume declines. This means that we are less and less able to pump oxygen and nutrient-rich blood to our working muscles during extended exertion.

Some of this decline is inevitable with age, but just as with loss of strength, bone density, and balance, much of the problem is self-inflicted through an excessively sedentary lifestyle. A targeted and appropriately calibrated aerobic exercise program can not only slow the onset of cardiovascular decline but also reverse it.[9]

According to the latest recommendations from the American College of Sports Medicine (ACSM), adults should get at least two and a half hours of moderate-intensity cardiorespiratory exercise per week. This goal can be met through 30–60 minutes of moderate-intensity exercise five days per week or 20–60 minutes of vigorous-intensity exercise three days per week, conducted in continuous daily sessions or broken up throughout the day in blocks of at least 10 minutes.[10]

Of course, if you're deconditioned and are not currently engaged in an exercise program, ACSM recommends that you build up gradually toward meeting these goals, slowly increasing the time, frequency, and intensity of your cardio exercise in order to avoid injury. After all, the point of exercise it to protect ourselves from injury and decline, not cause it.

This book is about strength training, but cardio exercise is also a crucial part of good health and should not be ignored. Remember, even if you are unable to meet the minimum ACSM recommendations for cardio exercise, *any* movement is better than no movement.

As a general goal, you should be doing some kind of movement that stresses your cardiovascular system every day. This doesn't mean that you have to train every day; you should just be active and move. So walking, mowing the lawn, and cycling to run errands all count. As far as strenuous cardio workouts are concerned, you should aim to do three workouts a week of at least 30 minutes duration each.

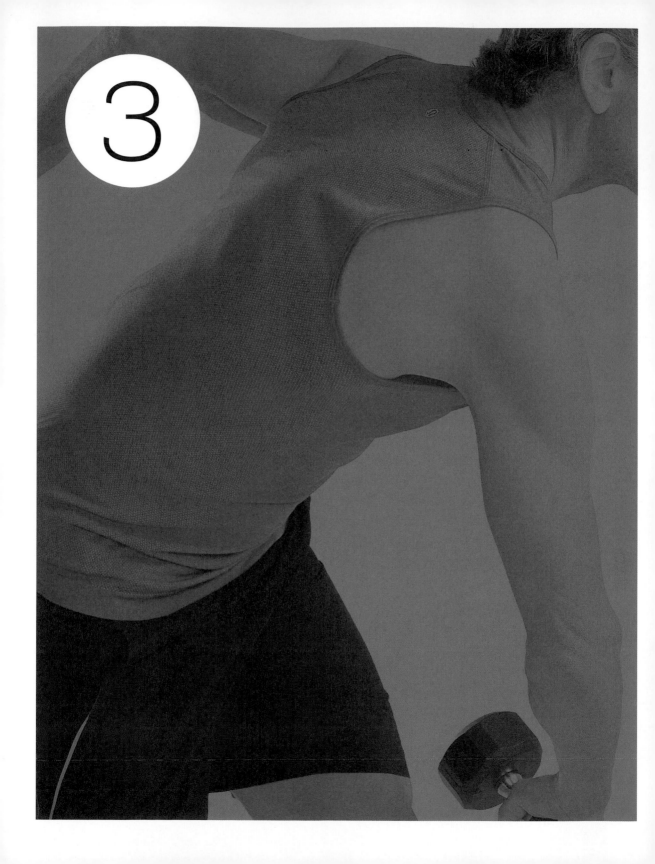

YOUR BODY, YOUR EQUIPMENT

In the previous two chapters we learned the ways in which our bodies prefer to move and the challenges that we face as we age. Now we can begin to use those insights from Chapter 1 to meet the challenges outlined in Chapter 2. In doing so, we'll progress from the theoretical to the practical, and introduce specific exercises and workouts to build improved health and fitness.

The first thing we'll need in order to accomplish this is a good working knowledge of our anatomy. Then we'll discuss the equipment needed to get started.

MEET YOUR MUSCLES

The human body contains three types of muscles: cardiac, smooth, and skeletal. There's really only one cardiac muscle—the heart. Smooth muscles are the muscles of our organs. Both are vitally important muscle groups, but we're going to ignore them here. In this chapter, we're interested only in skeletal muscles. They move bone and thereby help us perform work and achieve movement.

There are some 640 skeletal muscles in the human body, but that's a misleading number. Many of these are tiny muscles in our face that help us form expressions and move our eyes and tongue. Take these away, and we are left with about 400 muscles.

We can chop that number in half because each muscle is part of a pair. One is the agonist, or moving, muscle, and the other is the antagonist, or opposing, muscle. To perform any movement, the agonist muscle has to contract and thereby move the bone to which it's attached. The antagonist muscle must relax to permit the contraction. Otherwise, the two muscles create a stalemate.

Here's an example of how these pairs function. Consider a biceps dumbbell curl. To perform that exercise, you hold a dumbbell palm up and flex your elbow, raising the dumbbell toward your shoulder. This movement requires you to contract the biceps muscle. But in order to bend the elbow, the triceps muscle on the back of your arm has to relax and stretch.

Understanding pairing is important. This key concept will help organize our workouts: Whenever one muscle is working, its opposing muscle is resting. Put that in your back pocket for now; we'll return to it later.

So, we're now left with about 200 pairs of muscles. But even that list can be chopped down significantly because we organize many of these muscles into groups that together power the movements we will be performing. For example, there are four large muscles that together are referred to as the quadriceps group, found on the front of the upper leg. This muscle group powers extension of the knee. These muscles are opposed by three large muscles referred to as the hamstrings, located on the back of the leg, which powers flexion of the knee.

These groupings can be found all over the body, from the shoulders to the calves. Now we're getting to a manageable list of muscles.

The diagrams on pages 34 and 35, showing key muscle groups, have been organized further by collecting these groups of muscles into mega-groups that work together to perform big movements. This takes us down to just four categories:

1. **Push muscles:** The muscle groups of the chest, shoulders, and triceps, which help the body extend the arms and push the body away from something or push something away from the body.

2. **Pull muscles:** The muscle groups of the upper back and biceps, which together pull the body up or forward, or pull something down or toward the body.

3. **Rotation muscles:** The muscle groups of the torso, which power twisting movements. These include some of the core muscles discussed in the section on balance in Chapter 2.

4. **Leg muscles:** We'll collect all of the leg muscles together because many big leg movements involve all of the major muscle groups found here, including the legs' pushing and pulling muscles.

Although a given exercise may not use all of the muscles in the group in which its target muscle is located, it will certainly use at least some of them. For example, a dumbbell chest press uses all of the push muscles (chest, shoulders, and triceps), while a dumbbell shoulder press uses two of them (the shoulders and triceps).

Now let's return to the pairing concept discussed earlier. If an exercise uses one of the big muscle groups—the push muscles, for example—then the opposing muscles—the pull muscles—would not be working as hard. So when the primary muscle group being worked reaches temporary failure (the state at which it is too fatigued to do another repetition at that resistance level without resting first), the opposing muscle group is still fresh enough to get started on another exercise.

Is this a foolproof, comprehensive way to categorize exercises? No, for two reasons. First, although the concept of agonist and antagonist muscle groups teaches that one group is working while the opposing group is resting, the antagonist is never entirely quiet while the agonist is busy. That's because its job is to oppose the movement slowly and help control it so nothing gets damaged in the process.

To understand this, imagine a group of workers lowering a piano from a high floor using a rope and pulley. Even though they would rely on gravity to pull the piano down to street level, they would still be working quite hard to make sure it came down gently, and not with a piano-splitting crash. The same is true for your antagonist muscles.

The second reason the pairing concept is not watertight is that some exercises use muscle groups from two, three, or even all four of these categories. In fact, since movement complexity is one of our goals, we'll aim to accomplish exactly that.

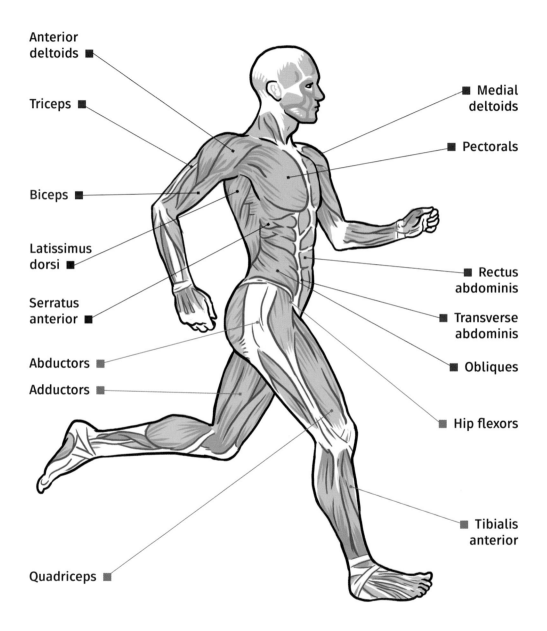

Anterior deltoids ■

Triceps ■

Biceps ■

Latissimus dorsi ■

Serratus anterior ■

Abductors ■

Adductors ■

Quadriceps ■

■ Medial deltoids

■ Pectorals

■ Rectus abdominis

■ Transverse abdominis

■ Obliques

■ Hip flexors

■ Tibialis anterior

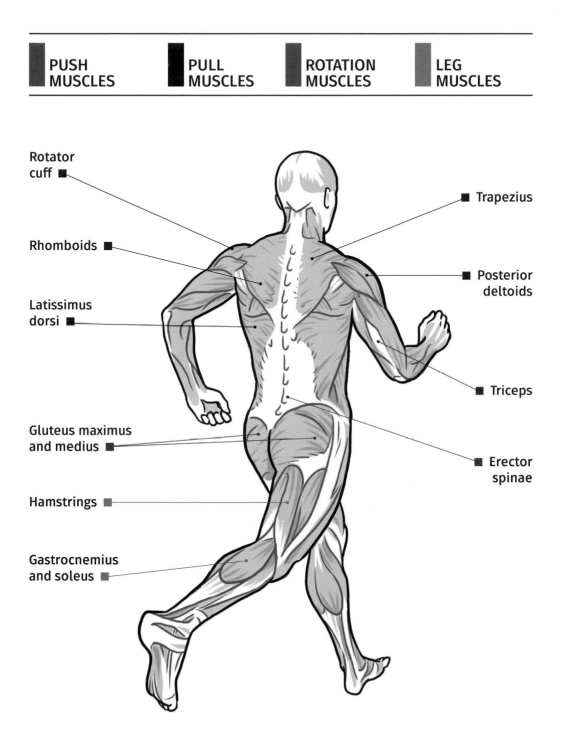

PUSH
MUSCLES

PULL
MUSCLES

ROTATION
MUSCLES

LEG
MUSCLES

Rotator
cuff

Rhomboids

Latissimus
dorsi

Gluteus maximus
and medius

Hamstrings

Gastrocnemius
and soleus

Trapezius

Posterior
deltoids

Triceps

Erector
spinae

So rather than thinking of the pairing framework as a law, think of it as a general guideline. It might not always provide an accurate description of a given exercise, but having this structure in mind will help us understand something important about each movement that we'll be doing.

MEET YOUR GYM

You may belong to an expensive state-of-the-art gym. In that case, the world is your oyster, and I encourage you to make good use of all the great equipment and services that your gym provides. But if you don't belong to a gym, or you belong to one but you can't seem to find the time to go there frequently, don't worry. The program presented in this book can be followed using a minimal amount of equipment. You can do it in the gym, but you can also do it at home with only a relatively small investment. Here's what you'll need.

YOURSELF

In many of our exercises, your body weight will provide all of the resistance you'll need. The movements that we'll do will strengthen your stabilizers and core muscles to improve your balance and ability to perform functional movements. In other words, you'll practice moving your body so that you become better at moving your body.

FREE WEIGHTS

For some exercises, your body weight alone doesn't provide enough of a challenge to bring about improvement. We'll need to increase the challenge by adding resistance. This is where free weights come in. The name *free weights* derives from the fact that these weights are not tethered to a cable or stacked in an exercise machine. This class of equipment includes barbells, dumbbells, kettlebells, and medicine balls. Typically, the price of the equipment depends on its weight, so the heavier the piece of equipment, the more expensive it will be.

I recommend investing in sets of dumbbells of various weight levels, since the

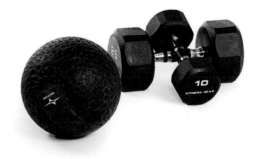

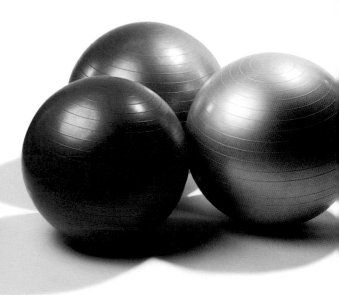

exercises that we'll be doing will recruit different muscles, and these muscles vary in the loads they can safely handle. Three pairs of dumbbells—light, medium, and heavy—will do the trick. I also recommend that you invest in a medicine ball of medium to heavy weight. It will be used both for resistance and as a tool to challenge other muscles as we scale exercises, making them more challenging.

STABILITY BALL

We will perform exercises with this large inflated ball and also use it as a platform to perform exercises on. Stability balls come in different sizes, and although manufacturers encourage you to buy the one corresponding to your height, I've found that the size of the ball doesn't really make a big difference in how you use it. Generally, I prefer the larger ones.

The variance in price among stability balls usually has to do with the thickness and durability of the plastic. The heavier the grade, the more you'll be able to inflate it, which will help with its performance. There's a noticeable difference between the top brands and the lesser brands, so choose the more durable brands if possible.

BOSU

This piece of equipment looks like a stability ball cut in half and mounted on a hard plastic base. Its purpose is to provide an unstable platform for your exercises, which forces your core and neuromuscular network to engage in order to keep you from falling. This leads to improvements in your balance and functional strength. Its name is an acronym for "Both Sides Up," which refers to its usefulness in both the soft side down and hard side down positions.

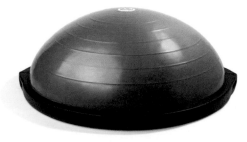

AB WHEEL

This deceptively simple-looking piece of equipment is just a wheel threaded through with an axle on which hand-grips have been mounted. It looks like it wouldn't do much, but in fact it can be devilishly hard to use and extremely effective. Best of all, it's inexpensive, lightweight, and travels well, making it one of the most efficient—and underappreciated—exercise tools ever invented.

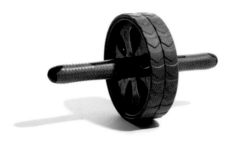

WORKOUT SPACE

Perhaps the most important piece of workout equipment you'll use is the floor upon which you'll be exercising. Most of the exercises presented here don't require a lot of room to perform, and because you won't be using big, heavy equipment, you won't need to dedicate any space to your workouts full time. You can get by with a space as small as 10 feet by 4 feet.

The surface of your workout space will affect your ability to do some of these exercises. Since many of them require you to lie on the floor, a hard surface will make performing these exercises uncomfortable or impossible. Aim to use a padded or carpeted area, if available, and further cushion it with a yoga mat or thin foam sleeping pad.

Some fitness experts will tell you to avoid distractions in your workout space, but I believe that things are a distraction only when you let them be a distraction. As long as you can concentrate on the exercises and not take any unnecessary breaks, I'll leave it to you to decide if you'd feel more motivated with the TV on or music playing in the background. But cell phones are different because answering a text or an email message often devolves into a trip down the proverbial rabbit hole. In my view, everyone is entitled to 30 minutes or so of free time, so unless it's a certifiable emergency, connect after your workout is over.

Now you know how your body works, what the challenges are, what you'll need to work out, and where you should work out. The foundation is complete. We're ready to talk about your program.

WHAT'S THE DEAL WITH STRETCHING?

Many people assume that stretching should play a role in our regular exercise routine. But the decision to stretch isn't necessarily a no-brainer. Here's why.

Strength is produced through the storage and release of tension in the muscles. Any reduction of this tension also reduces the amount of power that can be stored and released. Just as a rubber band doesn't work well when it gets stretched out, our muscles don't deliver much power if they are stretched and relaxed.

This is exactly what happens in the moments immediately following stretching. This, therefore, is a reasonable argument against stretching before exercise or strenuous activity. But what about stretching after an activity? That would still be helpful, right?

The answer is a definitive maybe. Studies have failed to show the expected decline in injuries or gains in performance that post-workout stretching would be expected to produce. But that doesn't mean stretching is bad for you or that you shouldn't do it. Most physical therapists and fitness professionals continue to recommend stretching to maintain a full range of motion throughout the body.

I agree with this consensus. Even if we can't prove how stretching helps, it is usually required for recovery of injured areas, and it certainly feels good. But there's an important question to ask when you find yourself feeling tight in a particular muscle group. Rather than simply assuming that you should stretch more, ask yourself why this tightness has occurred. More times than not, it is due to a strength imbalance that has put stress on a particular area, resulting in overuse and tightness. In this case, the ideal solution is not stretching alone, which can relieve that tightness temporarily, but also adjusting your exercise routine to improve balance among muscle groups, which helps reduce tightness in the long term.

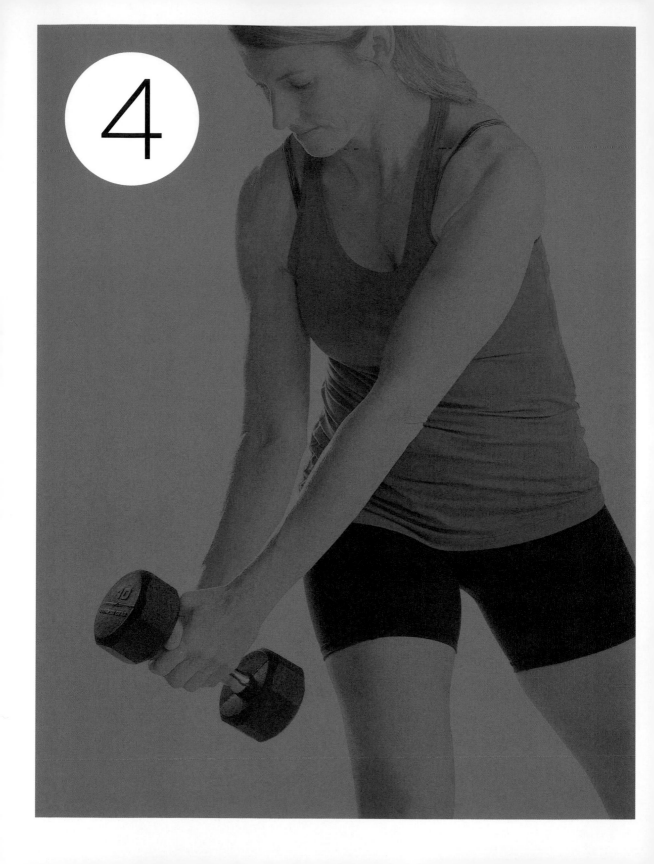

THE PROGRAM

I once had a training partner who approached her workouts like a kid going wild in a candy shop. For me, this was both a blessing and a curse, because while her enthusiasm and joy were infectious, her haphazard and chaotic approach to workouts left me frustrated and annoyed.

My friends and family might say I had this reaction because I have a controlling personality, a sometimes-unreasonable need to bring order to everything around me. That might be so. But still, I think that my reaction in that case was justified. Anyone working out should be able to articulate a rationale for what they're doing and how a particular workout fits into their overall fitness plan. If they can't articulate a reason for doing an exercise or routine, they shouldn't be doing it.

It isn't that every workout needs to be completely regimented, measured, and calibrated, or that movement for its own sake is useless. But for the best results and the most efficient use of time, a structured program that's based on a strong, rational foundation of applied theory is much more likely to get you where you want to go.

In this chapter we'll be discussing three things:

- The elements that comprise a complete strength training workout
- How *Ageless Strength* presents exercises in a way that incorporates those elements
- How to use this book to create complete workouts in a nearly endless variety

If you're worried that you are ill equipped to prepare your own workouts, don't be. In Chapter 6, I offer several exercise progressions to get you started and keep you going. You can use these as your go-to workouts, or use them as examples of what a workout should look like when you build your own routine. In either case, by the end of this chapter you'll be able to explain why you're doing a particular workout and how it's moving you closer to your goals.

THE ELEMENTS OF A COMPLETE WORKOUT

A good workout is like a delicious, balanced meal. Every item fits into the whole, bringing something new to the table that's neither redundant nor superfluous. And just like a good meal, each element of a workout not only contributes to your health but also makes the whole workout more interesting and enjoyable.

If this sounds too good to be true, that's because we've come to expect too little of our workouts. They are often treated like necessary evils, swallowed like bitter medicine that must be endured because it's good for us. The blame for bad workouts shouldn't be on the exercises themselves, but rather on program designers who fail to make the workouts varied and engaging. *Ageless Strength* works to amend that problem.

But let's be clear. Although the workouts in this book are designed to be fun and appealing, they are not a cakewalk. And that's as it should be. They will challenge you to improve, and thus they will involve some difficulty and require focus and persistence. But they will also reward you with a sense of satisfaction and accomplishment when you conquer them, especially as you mark your improvement over time.

The essential elements of these workouts should not be a surprise to you, because they address the three key challenges discussed in Chapter 2:

Balance: Exercises that increase your ability to control your body in space and keep it from falling, both in static positions and as you move.

Strength: Exercises that increase your ability to perform work, which is defined as exerting power over distance against resistance. These exercises provide stimuli to trigger an adaptive response that retains and improves muscular strength and bone density.

Functional: Exercises that involve applied strength and balance to perform movements that mimic the way the body moves in real life. These exercises prepare you for shoveling snow, storing boxes on the top shelves of your closet, and lifting heavy grocery bags and suitcases. In sum, this is where exercise meets the road and helps us through our daily lives.

A complete training program should contain exercises that address each of these elements, challenging you to improve balance, strength, and functionality with every workout, just as every meal should contain a carbohydrate, a protein, and a fat.

Many workout programs address at least one of the three. Some address two. A few address all three, but seldom in the same workout, and not consistently. This failure leaves a gap in your fitness regimen that can make you vulnerable to serious problems.

For example, if you work on improving strength by regularly doing bench presses and using the rowing machine, that will help you retain muscle mass and bone density but it won't help you keep your balance while walking on an icy road. Alternatively, practicing tai chi might help your balance, but it won't help prevent brittleness of your bones.

For many people, the challenge in structuring an effective workout program, or just knowing what program to follow, is identifying what benefit each exercise offers. If you don't know the benefits of the exercises you're doing, how do you know that you've done all that you could or should do to meet your goals?

This book ends that problem with a clear, easy-to-follow color-coding method. Exercises in the workout programs are organized under the following categories, which highlight the central ways in which they will challenge you:

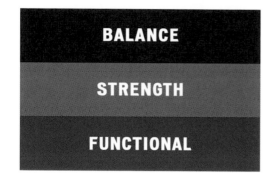

With that in mind, how do we go about building a workout? To illustrate, let's continue with our meal analogy. Imagine the list of exercises is like a dinner buffet. Each category—balance, strength, and functional—offers a number of exercises to choose from. But just as you would not eat every dish on a buffet in a single meal, you will not perform every listed exercise in a single workout. That would be counterproductive, since performing so many exercises in one workout could easily put too much stress on your body and lead to injury. At the very least, it would feel overwhelming and leave you unenthusiastic about your next workout.

Instead, you will sample from the exercises listed, trying a few from each category. On a buffet, it's simple work to identify the pasta, the meat, and the vegetables. Now, with our color-coding, it's just as easy to identify balance, strength, and functional exercises.

You may be able to handle some exercises with ease. Others will be very challenging. Although it might be tempting to perform only those exercises that you're comfortable with, that would be a mistake. Don't shy away from any of them. We all have a relative weakness in at least one of these categories. The point of our workouts is not to improve those areas in which we're already strong, it's to improve our conditioning in our weaker areas so that weaknesses become strengths and overall health and fitness improves.

In the workout progressions in Chapter 6, you'll see that each workout contains exercises from each category. As you go through the program, the number of exercises from each category increases from workout to workout. Like a plane taking off, we'll build our workouts as our fitness improves until we reach cruising altitude. At that time, we'll level off at 28–30 exercises in each workout. Our focus will then shift from increasing the volume of exercises to increasing the difficulty of the routine by arranging the exercises in more challenging ways.

In Chapter 7 we'll talk about where you can go with your training routine once you successfully complete the programs presented in Chapter 6. Before we can do that, however, let's get familiar with the exercises themselves.

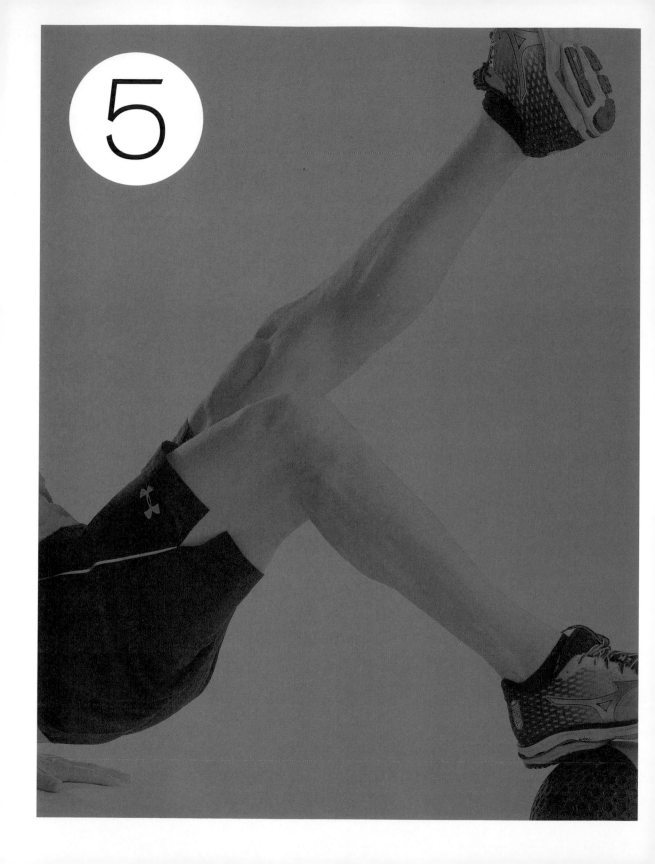

THE
EXERCISES

The exercises in this book are color-coded as balance ( ), strength ( ), and functional ( ). Each exercise designates one of these categories as its primary benefit. Many of these exercises have a broader benefit, however, and fall into two or more categories. For example, the push-up is coded blue, as a strength exercise. But it can also be considered a functional exercise because it challenges the core muscles. In addition, it engages your stabilizing muscles, especially in some of the more advanced and exotic variations, so it can be considered a balance exercise.

Though an exercise may have multiple designations, each is labeled for its primary characteristic. You can think of its other defining characteristics as additional benefits. So when you do a push-up, you are building strength, but if you feel your core being engaged or your balance being challenged, all the better.

Many exercises require you to perform repetitions on one side of the body and then the other. Make sure that you perform the exercise on both sides of the body. In some of the routines that you'll find later in the book, you may be instructed to perform another exercise before switching to the other side; this arrangement allows for better flow from movement to movement so that you won't simply rotate from one side to the other. Don't let these arrangements confuse you— you'll still work both sides of the body.

As I compiled these exercises and wrote down instructions, I was reminded of a popular piece of home exercise equipment from years ago. It resembled a child's hobbyhorse, and you rode it to improve your fitness. A least, that's how it was supposed to work. The problem was that the equipment used a person's own body weight as resistance. That meant that as a person became more fit and lost excess weight, the exercise got easier and easier because the resistance was continually reduced. To paraphrase Yogi Berra, the machine was so effective that eventually everyone stopped using it.

The takeaway lesson here is that to be useful for the long term, an exercise has to be scalable and responsive. If it's too difficult in the beginning, no one will start doing it, and if it becomes too easy later on, everyone will stop doing it.

To keep the workouts in this book sustainable for the long haul, I offer three versions of each exercise: a Level 1 version for beginners, a Level 2 version that's more challenging, and an advanced Level 3 version for those people who are ready to push themselves still further.

These designations are for ease of use, but don't feel stuck in them. Your choice of difficulty should take into account the other exercises that you'll be doing in that workout. For example, you might decide to put an easier exercise between two challenging ones in order to give yourself a bit of a breather. We'll discuss this more in Chapter 7, where you'll receive guidance on designing your own workouts. But for now, you should consider all of the exercise variations listed in this chapter as viable options.

As you review these exercises, you will see that I've listed the primary muscles worked along with the secondary muscles worked. As we've discussed, it's rare for the body to perform a movement using only one or two muscles. Although any given movement will place more of a burden on one particular muscle group than on others, it's much more efficient to get more muscle groups involved so they can share the burden.

By listing the secondary muscle groups, I hope to offer you a better understanding of how your body works and help you develop an appreciation for the complexity of these movements and your body's ability to perform them.

You'll notice that the transverse abdominis is listed as a secondary muscle group in many of these exercises. In truth, the transverse abdominis is engaged in almost all movement and thus in virtually every exercise listed here. However, I've highlighted it particularly in those exercises that require balance, since balance engages the transverse abdominis to an even greater degree that warrants special attention.

Note also that when an exercise is described as engaging your lateral stabilizers, this refers primarily to your transverse abdominis and your obliques. If you are standing, it also includes your gluteus medius, abductor, and adductor muscles.

Before you move on to the workouts provided in Chapter 6, I strongly suggest that you read through this section and become familiar with the movements. Practice them until you feel comfortable with at least the Level 1 form of each exercise. If you feel competent with that, try Level 2. Remember, there's no set timetable for fitness and health. Move along at your own pace, and don't rush your progress.

As with any exercise program, talk with your doctor before trying the movements and routines here. This is especially true if you have had any injuries that might limit your range of motion or if you take any medication that could affect your ability to perform these movements. As I tell all of my clients and training teams, our goal is to be smarter than we are brave. Forcing yourself through an exercise that you shouldn't be doing can lead to injury. That completely undermines the goal of this book.

Train with enthusiasm, train with focus, train with energy and commitment, but above all, train with intelligence.

BALANCE

52 Pistol Squats

54 One-Legged Deadlifts

56 Side Leg Swings

58 Front Leg Swings

60 Standing Hurdles

62 Reverse Hurdles

64 Military Sit-Ups

66 Leg Crossovers

68 Flutter Kicks

70 Knee Tucks

72 Stability Ball Leg Curls

74 Supine Plank with Leg Raises

76 Side Hip Raises

78 Reverse Leg Raises

80 V Sit-Ups

82 Russian Twists

84 Dumbbell Stability Ball Flyes

86 Side Knee Crunches

PISTOL SQUATS

Also called one-legged squats, this exercise is a good test of balance, but it also requires strength.

THE MOVEMENT

Stand on your right foot, holding your left leg out in front of you as straight as possible. Squat down as low as you comfortably can, and then rise back up. This constitutes 1 repetition (rep).

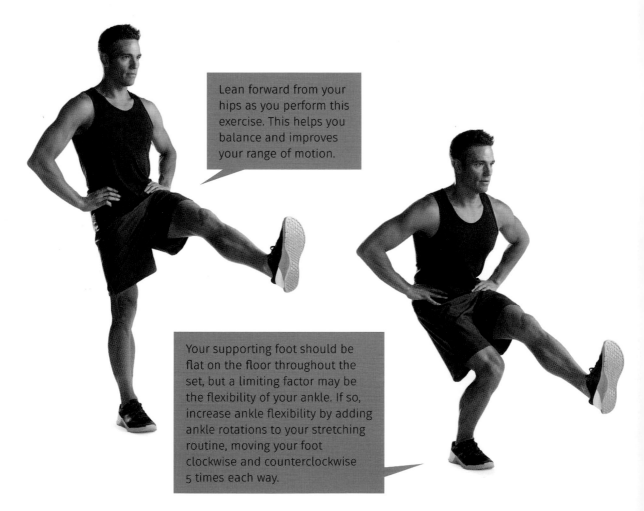

Lean forward from your hips as you perform this exercise. This helps you balance and improves your range of motion.

Your supporting foot should be flat on the floor throughout the set, but a limiting factor may be the flexibility of your ankle. If so, increase ankle flexibility by adding ankle rotations to your stretching routine, moving your foot clockwise and counterclockwise 5 times each way.

PRIMARY MUSCLES WORKED

▸ Quadriceps
▸ Hamstrings
▸ Gluteus maximus
▸ Gluteus medius

SECONDARY MUSCLES WORKED

▸ Transverse abdominis
▸ Erector spinae

◀ LEVEL **1**

Perform **THE MOVEMENT** as described.

LEVEL **2** ▸

Perform this exercise while holding a light dumbbell or medicine ball with both arms straight out in front of you (as shown). This shifts your center of gravity forward, which engages and challenges your lower back.

LEVEL **3**

Perform this exercise while standing on the soft side of a BOSU. This is a very challenging form of this movement. If you have difficulty, try doing only 1 or 2 squats, and then step off the BOSU and continue your set on solid ground. Aim to eventually complete an entire set from atop the BOSU.

Keep your supporting leg straight in front of you, drifting neither inward nor outward as you perform this exercise. Lateral drift indicates that either your adductor muscles or your abductor and outer hip muscles are overpowering their counterparts. If this describes your pistol squat, stretch the muscle group on the side that is pulling and work on strengthening the opposite muscles.

ONE-LEGGED DEADLIFTS

This exercise is called a deadlift because it places your upper body in an unsupported cantilever position, which engages your lower back. It's also a great balance and flexibility exercise.

THE MOVEMENT

Stand on your left foot and bend your left knee slightly to engage the muscles of the planted leg. Bend over as far as you can while raising your right leg high in the air behind you. Keep your body and raised leg in a straight line. Continue until your body is parallel to the floor, and then return to a standing position. This constitutes 1 rep.

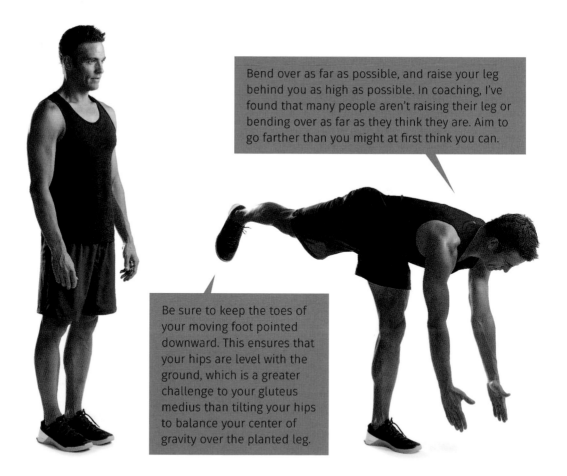

Bend over as far as possible, and raise your leg behind you as high as possible. In coaching, I've found that many people aren't raising their leg or bending over as far as they think they are. Aim to go farther than you might at first think you can.

Be sure to keep the toes of your moving foot pointed downward. This ensures that your hips are level with the ground, which is a greater challenge to your gluteus medius than tilting your hips to balance your center of gravity over the planted leg.

PRIMARY MUSCLES WORKED

▶ Erector spinae
▶ Hamstrings

SECONDARY MUSCLES WORKED

▶ Gluteus medius
▶ Transverse abdominis

LEVEL 1

Perform **THE MOVEMENT** as described.

LEVEL 2 ▶

Hold a light medicine ball or dumbbell with both hands in front of you (as shown). This helps you maintain balance, as the weight acts like ballast on a ship. It also increases the challenge to your lower back, which will need to counter the pull of the extra resistance.

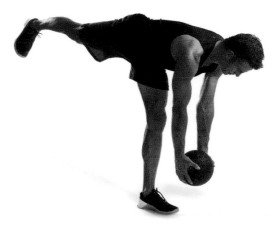

LEVEL 3

Perform this movement while standing on the soft side of a BOSU. This is very challenging, so don't rush the movement and don't be discouraged if you have difficulty with it at first.

SIDE LEG SWINGS

This is a balance exercise that also serves to stretch and strengthen the outer hip.

THE MOVEMENT

Stand straight with hands on your hips and your right leg positioned across your midline. Swing that leg out to the side as high as you can, and then swing it back across your midline like a pendulum. This constitutes 1 rep.

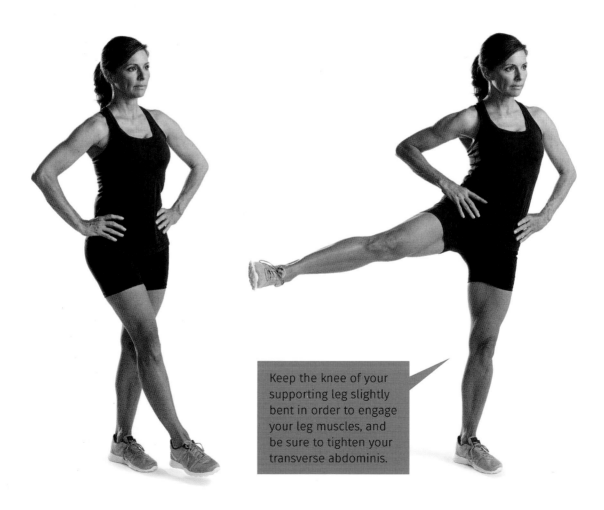

Keep the knee of your supporting leg slightly bent in order to engage your leg muscles, and be sure to tighten your transverse abdominis.

PRIMARY MUSCLES WORKED

▸ Gluteus medius

SECONDARY MUSCLES WORKED

▸ Transverse abdominis
▸ Adductors
▸ Abductors
▸ Calf muscles
  (in advanced form)

◀ ## LEVEL **1**

Perform **THE MOVEMENT** as described.

LEVEL **2**

Perform this exercise with your eyes closed. Removing visual cues challenges your brain to rely more on your strength and proprioception.

LEVEL **3** ▶

Perform this exercise while standing on the soft side of a BOSU (as shown). This challenging form of the exercise requires you to hold your supporting ankle in a stable position, in addition to maintaining your balance as your swinging leg keeps shifting your center of gravity.

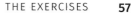

FRONT LEG SWINGS

This is a balance exercise that also serves to stretch and strengthen the hip flexors.

Standing on your left leg, swing your right leg behind you and then swing it forward as high as you comfortably can. This constitutes 1 rep. You can hold your arms still at your hips or swing them in opposition to your legs as if you were walking.

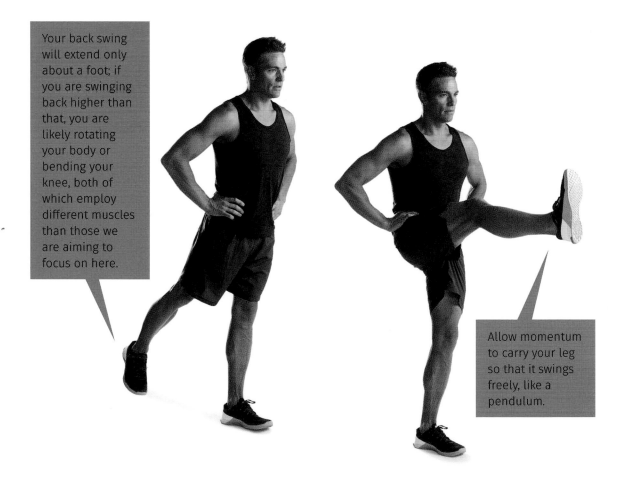

Your back swing will extend only about a foot; if you are swinging back higher than that, you are likely rotating your body or bending your knee, both of which employ different muscles than those we are aiming to focus on here.

Allow momentum to carry your leg so that it swings freely, like a pendulum.

PRIMARY MUSCLES WORKED

▶ Hip flexors

SECONDARY MUSCLES WORKED

▶ Transverse abdominis
▶ Quadriceps
▶ Gluteus maximus
▶ Calf muscles
  (in advanced form)

◀ LEVEL **1**

Perform **THE MOVEMENT** as described.

LEVEL **2**

Perform this exercise with your eyes closed. This removes visual cues from the data that your brain processes to maintain balance, and it forces your body to enhance its strength instead.

LEVEL **3** ▶

Perform this exercise while standing on the soft side of a BOSU (as shown). This increases the challenge by destabilizing your base, which requires your brain to figure out how to use your neuromuscular system to reestablish balance.

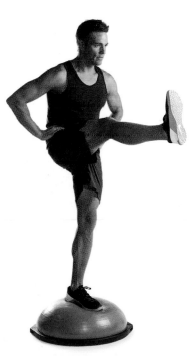

STANDING HURDLES

This exercise opens up your hip and increases flexibility in that area, but its equally important purpose is to improve your balance and strengthen your supporting muscles.

THE MOVEMENT

With hands on hips, stand on your left leg and bring your right knee up and out to the side. Keeping that knee bent, bring it forward, down, and back to the side, drawing a circle with the knee. This constitutes 1 rep.

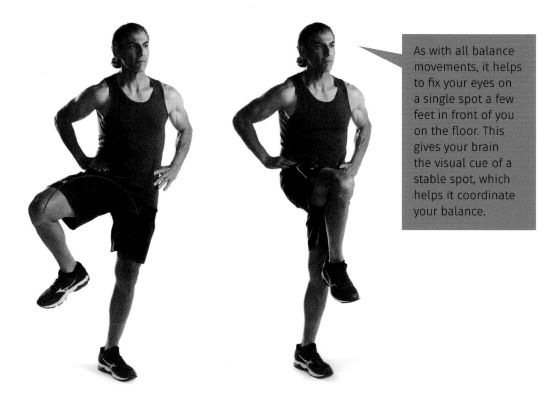

As with all balance movements, it helps to fix your eyes on a single spot a few feet in front of you on the floor. This gives your brain the visual cue of a stable spot, which helps it coordinate your balance.

PRIMARY MUSCLES WORKED

▸ Gluteus medius

SECONDARY MUSCLES WORKED

▸ Transverse abdominis
▸ Hip flexors
▸ Quadriceps
▸ Adductors
▸ Calf muscles
  (in advanced form)

◀ ## LEVEL **1**

Perform **THE MOVEMENT** as described.

LEVEL **2**

Perform this exercise with your eyes closed. This will remove visual cues from the data that your brain processes to maintain balance, and it will force your body to enhance your strength instead.

LEVEL **3** ▶

Perform this exercise while standing on the soft side of a BOSU (as shown). This destabilizes your base and requires your brain to figure out how to use your neuromuscular system to reestablish balance.

REVERSE HURDLES

This exercise performs the same function as the standing hurdles, but by going the opposite direction, it works the abductors (outer leg muscles) instead of the adductors (inner leg muscles). This constitutes 1 rep.

THE MOVEMENT

With hands on hips, stand on your left leg and bring your right knee up in front of you. Keep that knee bent, swing it out and down and back up, drawing a large circle with your knee. This constitutes 1 rep.

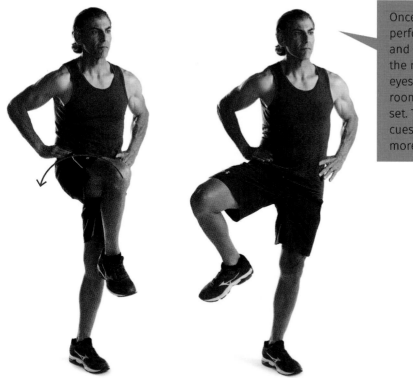

Once you are comfortable performing this exercise and feel stable throughout the movement, allow your eyes to wander around the room as you perform your set. This disrupts your visual cues, making this exercise more challenging.

**PRIMARY
MUSCLES WORKED**

▸ Gluteus medius

**SECONDARY
MUSCLES WORKED**

▸ Transverse abdominis
▸ Hip flexors
▸ Quadriceps
▸ Abductors
▸ Calf muscles
  (in advanced form)

◀ LEVEL **1**

Perform **THE MOVEMENT** as described.

LEVEL **2**

Perform this exercise with your eyes closed.

LEVEL **3** ▶

Perform this exercise while standing on the soft side of a BOSU (as shown). This destabilizes your base and requires your brain to figure out how to use your neuromuscular system to reestablish balance.

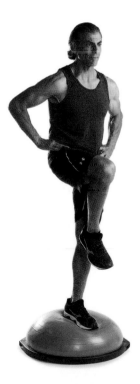

MILITARY SIT-UPS

These are like sit-ups, but with an additional challenge thrown in for the hip flexors and legs. In the advanced forms, it also engages your lateral stabilizers.

THE MOVEMENT

Sit on the floor (or on an exercise mat) with your hands on the floor behind you. Lean back far enough to be able to lift your legs off the floor straight out in front of you. Bring your knees to your chest, and then straighten your legs back out again, keeping your legs in the air throughout the movement. That's 1 rep. Especially as you get used to this movement, rest your feet on the floor between repetitions as necessary.

Keep your trunk as vertical as possible during this movement. Lying back provides a counterweight to your legs, so the more upright you sit, the more you are relying on muscle strength (not leverage) to keep your legs aloft.

Make sure that you focus more on drawing your knees to your chest than on bending your knees. We're concerned with hip flexors, not hamstrings, so what happens at the knee is less important than what happens at the hips. Sometimes people perform this exercise by simply bending and straightening their knees, and that won't work the muscles that you're aiming for with this exercise.

PRIMARY
MUSCLES WORKED

▶ Rectus abdominis
▶ Hip flexors

SECONDARY
MUSCLES WORKED

▶ Erector spinae
▶ Quadriceps
▶ Lateral stabilizers
  (in advanced forms)

LEVEL **1**

Perform **THE MOVEMENT** as described.

LEVEL **2**

Start with your hands behind your head instead of on the floor, balancing on your tailbone throughout the exercise.

LEVEL **3** ▶

Hold a light dumbbell in each hand, up and out to your sides, weights vertical (as shown). As you bring your knees to your chest, bring the dumbbells together in front of you. You won't be able to use very heavy weights, but that's okay. The point is not to challenge your chest and shoulder muscles as much as to challenge your body to recalculate its point of balance and engage your stabilizing muscles even more.

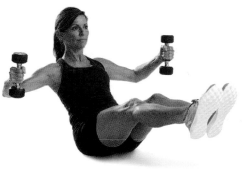

LEG CROSSOVERS

This exercise engages the lateral stabilizers, improves balance, works the inner and outer leg, and challenges the rest of the body to hold the position while you perform the movement. That's a lot of work in a single exercise!

THE MOVEMENT

Lean back, with palms on the ground behind you. With pointed toes, straighten your legs and lift them up off the ground in front of you. Spread them wide and then scissor them, alternating one leg over the other (that is, cross your right leg over your left, spread out wide, cross your left leg over your right leg, and so on). Crossing your right leg over your left and then your left leg over your right constitutes 1 rep.

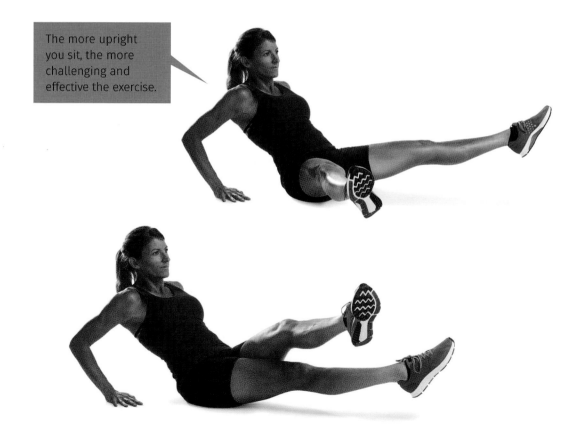

The more upright you sit, the more challenging and effective the exercise.

PRIMARY MUSCLES WORKED

▶ Abductors
▶ Adductors

LEVEL 1

Perform **THE MOVEMENT** as described.

LEVEL 2

Perform as described, but keep your hands off the floor, balancing entirely on your tailbone.

SECONDARY MUSCLES WORKED

▶ Gluteus medius
▶ Rectus abdominis
▶ Hip flexors
▶ Erector spinae
▶ Lateral stabilizers
▶ Transverse abdominis

LEVEL 3 ▶

Perform the movement while holding one dumbbell in one hand off to the side (as shown). The dumbbell doesn't have to be heavy. All we want is to put a little tug on one side of your body to force your core to compensate. This additional challenge will strengthen your stabilizing muscles.

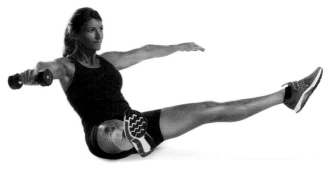

FLUTTER KICKS

This exercise primarily challenges the hip flexor muscles, but also engages a wide range of supportive and stabilizing muscles.

THE MOVEMENT

While balancing on your tailbone, stretch your legs out straight in front of you and lean back on your forearms. Alternate swinging each leg up and down, as if swimming. Keep your legs off the floor throughout the movement. Let your legs rest between sets if necessary. Fluttering your right leg and left leg up and down one time each constitutes 1 rep.

Feel free to flutter your arms in front of you in counterpoint to the movement of your legs (left leg and right arm, right leg and left arm, and so on).

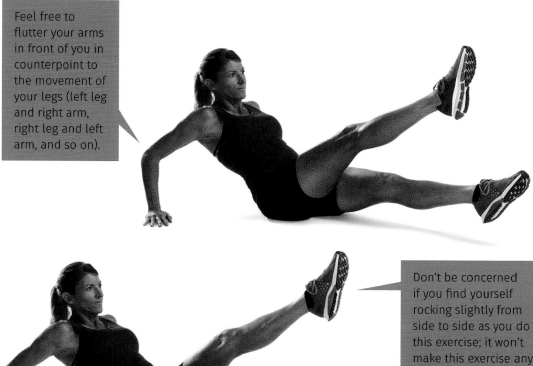

Don't be concerned if you find yourself rocking slightly from side to side as you do this exercise; it won't make this exercise any less effective. On the contrary, it might help you find a rhythm that makes completing the exercise easier.

PRIMARY MUSCLES WORKED

▶ Hip flexors
▶ Deltoids (in advanced form)

LEVEL **1**

Perform **THE MOVEMENT** as described.

LEVEL **2** ▶

Perform exercise as described, but hold your hands straight out in front of you or behind your head (as shown).

LEVEL **3**

Perform the exercise while holding light dumbbells straight out to your sides. This engages your deltoid muscles.

SECONDARY MUSCLES WORKED

▶ Rectus abdominis
▶ Quadriceps
▶ Erector spinae

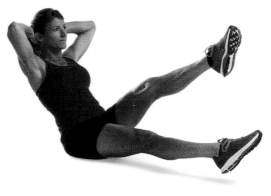

KNEE TUCKS

This exercise is harder than it looks, since it requires good upper body strength, core strength, and balance. Don't get discouraged if you have difficulty performing it initially; with practice, you'll get the hang of it. Even if you are great at performing push-ups, you may be surprised at the difficulty of the knee tuck. That's because of the great amount of time spent in a push-up position (also referred to as a plank position). In the time it takes to perform 1 knee tuck, you might be able to do 5 push-ups. So even those who can do a lot of push-ups might struggle to get through several of these movements.

THE MOVEMENT

Assume a push-up position, resting on your hands but placing your shins on a stability ball. Bend your knees and roll the ball toward your chest, then roll it out again until your legs are straight. This constitutes 1 rep.

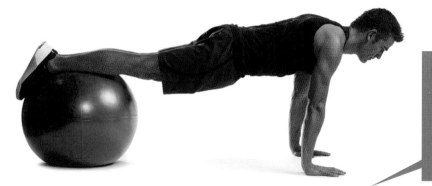

Avoid swinging your hips up and down as you perform this exercise. Your upper body should remain still throughout the movement.

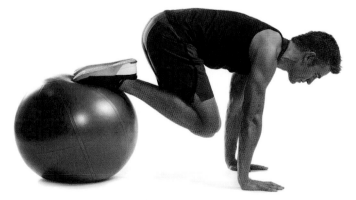

▸ Hip flexors

▸ Chest
▸ Deltoids
▸ Triceps
▸ Rectus abdominis
▸ Erector spinae
▸ Gluteus medius
▸ Transverse abdominis

◀ LEVEL **1**

Perform **THE MOVEMENT** as described. If this feels too challenging, drop onto your forearms. This eliminates your triceps from the exercise, as you will no longer have to work to keep your arms straight.

LEVEL **2**

To make this exercise more challenging, move the ball from your shins to the tops of your feet. Or better yet, move the ball onto your toes. The more of your body that you have on the stability ball, the more stable you will be, so the less of your body that touches the ball, the more you'll have to engage your stabilizing muscles to keep from rolling to the side and falling off.

LEVEL **3** ▶

To increase the challenge and to more actively engage some of the secondary muscles, perform a push-up between each repetition of knee tucks. Or, perform the tuck with your hands holding onto the sides of a BOSU (as shown).

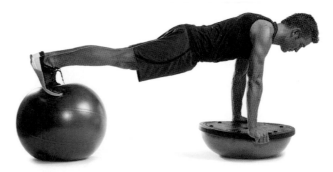

STABILITY BALL LEG CURLS

The main muscle group being worked in this one is the hamstrings, but many other muscles are engaged to hold your body in position while you perform the movement.

THE MOVEMENT

Lie on your back with your calves on the stability ball, arms spread out to the sides to remain stable. Raise your hips until your body is straight as a board from your shoulders to your feet. Bend your knees and roll the ball in toward your body, coming as close to touching your backside as possible. Roll the ball out again to the starting position. (If necessary, bend your elbows and use your hands to prop up your backside.) This constitutes 1 rep.

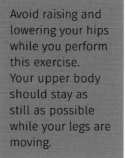

Avoid raising and lowering your hips while you perform this exercise. Your upper body should stay as still as possible while your legs are moving.

Note that the wider you spread your feet on the ball, the more control you have. Since we aim to destabilize the body as much as possible in order to work the core, as you grow stronger, work to keep your feet as close together as possible. And don't let your hips sag or rock up and down.

**PRIMARY
MUSCLES WORKED**

▶ Hamstrings

**SECONDARY
MUSCLES WORKED**

▶ Gluteus maximus
▶ Gluteus medius
▶ Erector spinae
▶ Hip flexors
▶ Transverse abdominis

◀ LEVEL **1**

Perform **THE MOVEMENT** as described.

LEVEL **2**

Bring your feet close together on the stability ball.
This limits your ability to triangulate between your
shoulders and your feet, reducing your points of
contact from three (shoulders and two separated
feet) to two (shoulders and two feet together).
This decrease in lateral stability makes your core
work harder.

LEVEL **3** ▶

For a real challenge, lie with your shoulders and upper
back on the soft side of a BOSU, with arms raised and
feet on the stability ball (as shown). This will leave you
without any contact with solid ground, thus forcing
your transverse abdominis to work harder to keep you
from tipping over.

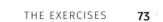

SUPINE PLANK WITH LEG RAISES

This exercise gauges your strength-to-weight ratio, since you have to be able to hold your body still in space and perform a difficult movement. You'll likely find this to be one of those exercises that's harder than it looks.

THE MOVEMENT

Sit on the floor with your heels on the floor, your knees partly bent, and your palms on the floor behind you. Raise your hips up so that you are resting only on your hands and heels. Raise your right leg as high as you can, keeping it as straight as you can, and lower it back down without letting it touch the floor. This constitutes 1 rep.

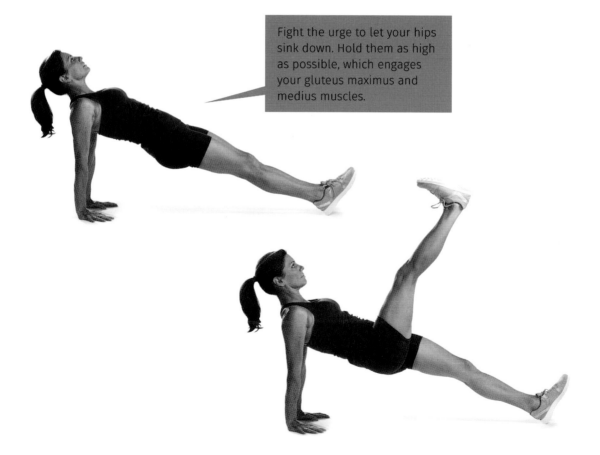

Fight the urge to let your hips sink down. Hold them as high as possible, which engages your gluteus maximus and medius muscles.

▸ Hip flexors
▸ Quadriceps
▸ Gluteus maximus
▸ Gluteus medius
▸ Erector spinae

▸ Deltoids
▸ Triceps

LEVEL **1**

To decrease the difficulty, do the exercise as described, but lower yourself down on your elbows and bend your knees more.

◀ LEVEL **2**

Perform **THE MOVEMENT** as described.

LEVEL **3** ▶

Place the heel of the supporting leg on the center of the soft side of a BOSU (as shown).

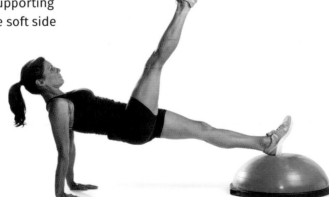

SIDE HIP RAISES

This exercise engages the oblique muscles, but in doing so it also challenges the outer hips as well as your sense of balance.

THE MOVEMENT

Lie on your side. Raise your hips in the air in a side plank position, holding your body in a rigid line from your feet to your shoulders while resting on your elbow. Lower your hips down—aim to avoid touching them to the floor—then raise them back up again. This constitutes 1 rep.

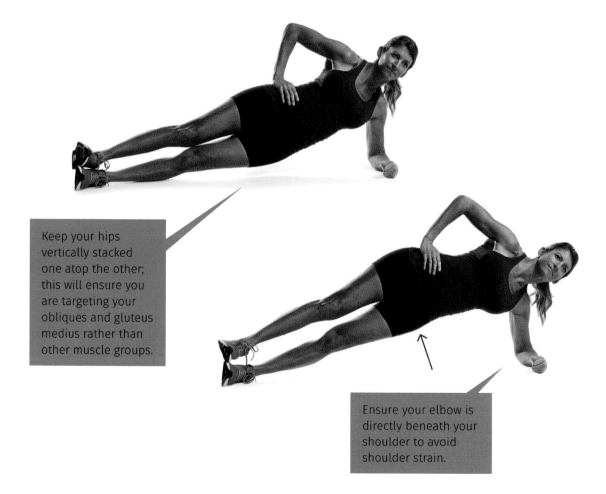

Keep your hips vertically stacked one atop the other; this will ensure you are targeting your obliques and gluteus medius rather than other muscle groups.

Ensure your elbow is directly beneath your shoulder to avoid shoulder strain.

PRIMARY MUSCLES WORKED

▸ Obliques
▸ Gluteus medius

SECONDARY MUSCLES WORKED

▸ Deltoids
▸ Transverse abdominis

◀ ## LEVEL **1**

Perform **THE MOVEMENT** as described. If necessary, place the palm of your top arm on the floor in front of you for balance.

LEVEL **2**

Start in a side plank position as in Level 1, but raise your top arm straight up in the air to decrease leverage and engage your stabilizing muscles further. Increase the challenge by holding a light dumbbell in that hand, and experiment by moving it to different positions.

LEVEL **3** ▶

Place your ankles on a BOSU, which destabilizes you and changes your position relative to gravity (as shown). You can also further engage the gluteus medius of the top hip by raising your top leg off your lower leg and holding it steady in the air as you perform this movement.

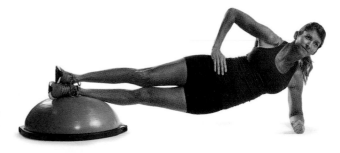

REVERSE LEG RAISES

Many of the exercises that we do engage the lower back and glutes as secondary muscles. This is one of the few that works these muscles directly.

THE MOVEMENT

Lie facedown on the stability ball with your palms on the floor. Roll forward until the ball is beneath your hips and your legs are in the air. Now raise your legs from your hips and lower them back down. This constitutes 1 rep.

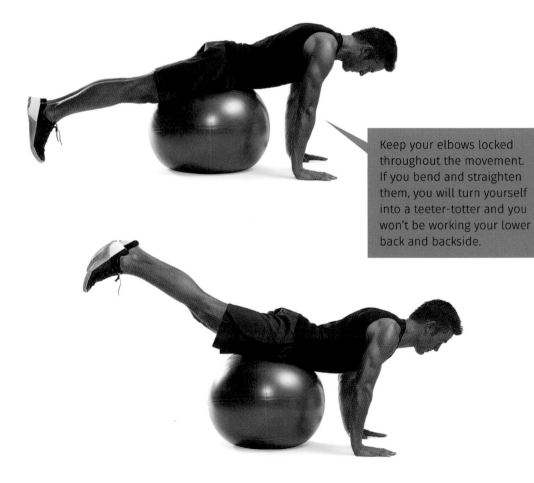

Keep your elbows locked throughout the movement. If you bend and straighten them, you will turn yourself into a teeter-totter and you won't be working your lower back and backside.

PRIMARY MUSCLES WORKED

▶ Erector spinae
▶ Gluteus maximus

SECONDARY MUSCLES WORKED

▶ Pectorals
▶ Deltoids
▶ Triceps

LEVEL 1

Perform the exercise as described, but roll forward so that the ball is beneath your body a bit lower. This provides more support for your lower body, making this exercise just a little bit easier to perform.

◀ LEVEL 2

Perform **THE MOVEMENT** as described. Your legs should be able to move freely without contacting the stability ball.

LEVEL 3 ▶

Add a BOSU, turning it soft side down and holding the front edge (as shown). Lift your legs. You will find that you have to work hard to keep the BOSU steady as you perform this movement.

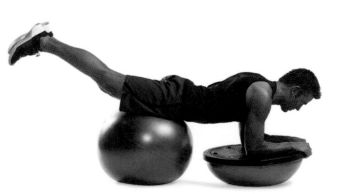

V SIT-UPS

This exercise is a double threat: It works the front abdominals while engaging the stabilizing muscles on the back of your body, all while challenging your brain to balance your body during the movement. No wonder it's such an effective exercise.

THE MOVEMENT

Start in a sitting position with your hands behind your head and legs stretched out in front of you. Raise your legs up together, and then lower them back down, almost to the floor. This constitutes 1 rep. Be sure to keep your knees extended throughout the exercise.

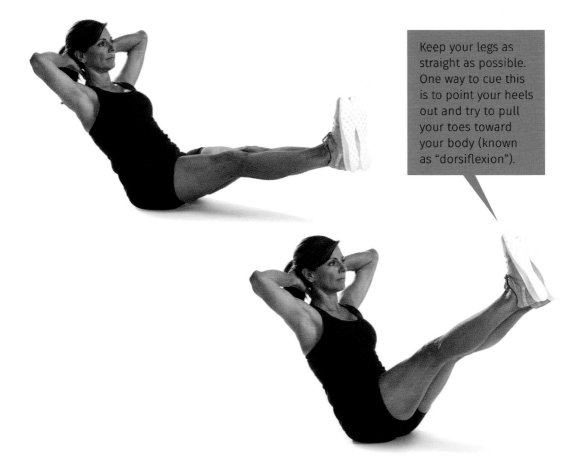

Keep your legs as straight as possible. One way to cue this is to point your heels out and try to pull your toes toward your body (known as "dorsiflexion").

**PRIMARY
MUSCLES WORKED**

▸ Rectus abdominis
▸ Hip flexors

**SECONDARY
MUSCLES WORKED**

▸ Erector spinae
▸ Quadriceps
▸ Transverse abdominis
▸ Obliques (in advanced
  form)

LEVEL **1**

Perform the exercise as described
but keep your palms on the ground
behind you throughout this exercise.
Leaning back while you perform this
exercise provides a counterweight
to your legs, giving you leverage to
balance. As you feel stronger, try
sitting more upright. This engages
your lower back and abdominal
muscles instead, and encourages
your body to adapt to this challenge.

◀ LEVEL **2**

Perform **THE MOVEMENT** as described.
You are balancing entirely on your
tailbone, which engages your
lower back.

LEVEL **3** ▶

Begin from the Level 2 starting
position, and turn this into a twisting
V sit-up by rotating your left elbow
toward your right leg on 1 repetition,
your right elbow toward your left leg
on the next, and so on (as shown).
This rotation engages your oblique
muscles in addition to everything
else you've been doing.

You may find yourself
rotating your legs and feet
in the opposite direction as
you rotate your upper body,
and that's perfectly fine.

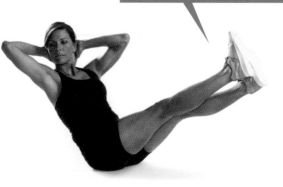

RUSSIAN TWISTS

This exercise involves rotation against resistance, and perhaps the biggest challenge is balancing on your tailbone as you twist and turn.

THE MOVEMENT

Sitting on the floor or an exercise mat, hold a dumbbell or medicine ball with both hands. Knees should be bent, with heels on the floor. Swing the weight to the right and then to the left. This constitutes 1 rep. You can also do this without a dumbbell as you focus on mastering the movement.

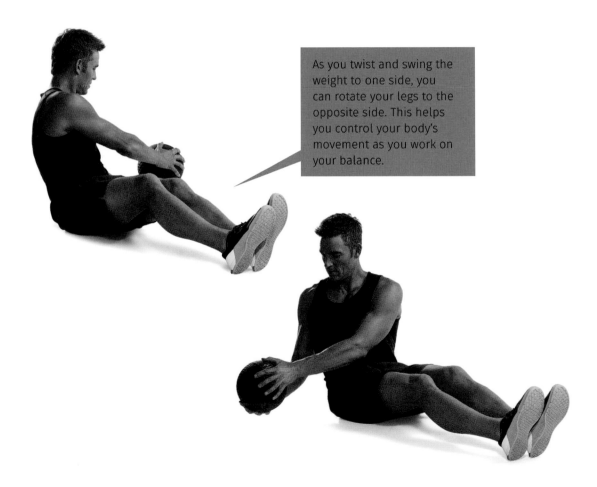

As you twist and swing the weight to one side, you can rotate your legs to the opposite side. This helps you control your body's movement as you work on your balance.

PRIMARY MUSCLES WORKED

▸ Obliques
▸ Deltoids

SECONDARY MUSCLES WORKED

▸ Transverse abdominis
▸ Erector spinae
▸ Rectus abdominis
  (in advanced form)

◀ LEVEL **1**

Perform **THE MOVEMENT** as described.

LEVEL **2** ▶

Do the exercise as described, but balance on your tailbone as you swing the weight to the right and then to the left. Allow your feet to rise off the ground (as shown); this will engage your lower rectus abdominis muscles.

LEVEL **3**

Use a heavier weight. This increases the centrifugal force of your rotation and challenges your obliques and transverse abdominis to stop the resulting momentum. It also increases the challenge to your arms and shoulders, which must work hard simply to hold the weight during the exercise.

DUMBBELL STABILITY BALL FLYES

This single-joint movement directly works your chest and front shoulders, but it also challenges your stabilizing muscles. So it's actually a balance exercise that's disguised as a strength exercise.

THE MOVEMENT

Lie back on a stability ball so that it is supporting your upper back, shoulders, and head. Grip a dumbbell in each hand and hold them directly overhead, slightly touching. With elbows slightly bent and pointing outward, spread your arms wide until you feel a stretch across your chest, and then bring your arms back to your starting position. This constitutes 1 rep.

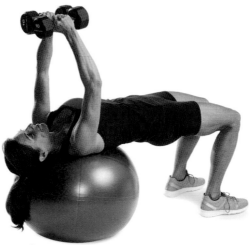

Ensure the ball is positioned so that your head is supported, to avoid neck strain. Remember to keep your elbows consistently bent throughout the movement. If you bend and then straighten your elbows, you will change this from a fly exercise to a press. A press introduces the triceps to the exercise, which makes it easier, thus reducing the challenge.

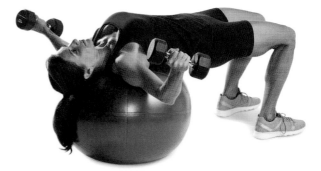

PRIMARY MUSCLES WORKED

▸ Pectorals
▸ Anterior deltoids

SECONDARY MUSCLES WORKED

▸ Transverse abdominis
▸ Erector spinae
▸ Gluteus maximus
▸ Gluteus medius

LEVEL **1**

Perform the exercise while lying on an exercise mat.

◂ ## LEVEL **2**

Perform **THE MOVEMENT** as described.

LEVEL **3** ▸

Perform the exercise by lying back on a stability ball while keeping your feet on the soft side of a BOSU (as shown). This destabilizes you further, requiring even more core stabilization. To increase the challenge, flip the BOSU so the soft side is facing down and your feet are on the hard side.

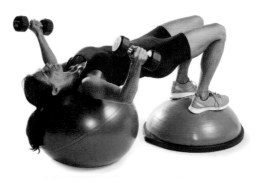

SIDE KNEE CRUNCHES

This movement engages your side abdominal muscles and works on balance as well. It also improves proprioception, as you get used to moving your body in a new way.

THE MOVEMENT

Lie on your side, propped up on one elbow, with your forearm on the floor. Raise your legs up off the ground, keeping them together with one leg stacked atop the other. Keeping your legs in the air, draw your knees in toward your chest, then push them back out again. This constitutes 1 rep.

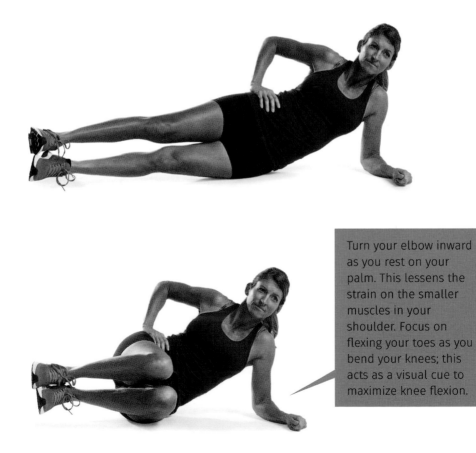

Turn your elbow inward as you rest on your palm. This lessens the strain on the smaller muscles in your shoulder. Focus on flexing your toes as you bend your knees; this acts as a visual cue to maximize knee flexion.

▸ Obliques
▸ Hip flexors
▸ Rectus abdominis

**SECONDARY
MUSCLES WORKED**

▸ Quadriceps
▸ Erector spinae
▸ Deltoids
▸ Triceps
▸ Transverse abdominis
  (in advanced forms)

◀ ## LEVEL **1**

Perform **THE MOVEMENT** as described. To increase the difficulty, lean on your palm rather than your elbow.

LEVEL **2**

Instead of lying on the floor, lie on the soft side of a BOSU with your palm on the floor behind you. This destabilizes you more, which further engages your transverse abdominis.

LEVEL **3** ▸

Lie on a BOSU as in Level 2, but instead of placing your palm on the floor behind you, put it directly on the BOSU, as shown. (Putting your hand behind you will give you greater stability, while moving forward will be more challenging.) Now you have no contact with solid ground, which challenges your brain to improve your balance.

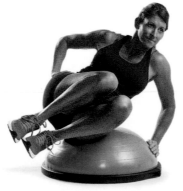

STRENGTH

90 Triceps Extensions

92 Lateral Raises

94 Front Raises

96 High Reverse Flyes

98 Low Reverse Flyes

100 Standing Shoulder Presses

102 Monkey Squats

104 Roll Outs

106 Roll Ups

108 Hip Thrusts

110 Push-Ups

112 Crunches

114 Crossover Crunches

116 Leg Raises

118 Fire Hydrants

120 Donkey Kicks

122 Supermans

124 Side Crunches

126 Side Leg Raises

128 Pullovers

130 Adductor Leg Raises

132 Windshield Wipers

TRICEPS EXTENSIONS

This exercise works the muscles on the back of your arms through elbow extension. By holding a weight high overhead, you are extending your body weight away from your center of gravity. This puts pressure on your core, challenging it and triggering positive adaptations.

THE MOVEMENT

Stand and hold a medium-weight dumbbell or a medicine ball overhead with both hands. Bend your elbows and lower the weight down behind your head, and then raise it back up again. This constitutes 1 rep.

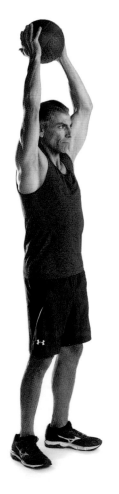

Keep your upper arms as close to the sides of your head and as still as possible. Aim to move only your forearms. This ensures that your triceps are doing most of the active work, as intended.

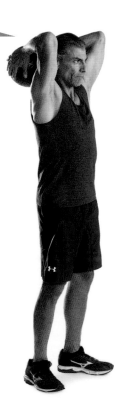

**PRIMARY
MUSCLES WORKED**

▸ Triceps

**SECONDARY
MUSCLES WORKED**

▸ Erector spinae
▸ Transverse abdominis
▸ Deltoids

◀ LEVEL **1**

Perform **THE MOVEMENT** as described.

LEVEL **2** ▶

Perform the exercise one arm at a time (as shown), using a lighter dumbbell or medicine ball than you would if you were using both hands. This increases the challenge to your shoulder muscles, as they work harder to balance the upraised arm.

LEVEL **3**

Perform half of the repetitions while standing on one leg, and then switch to the other leg. Start by holding a dumbbell or medicine ball with both hands, and when you feel competent with the movement, try doing it one arm at a time. Alternatively, stand on the soft side of a BOSU.

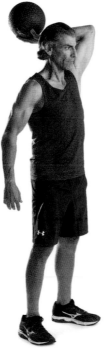

LATERAL RAISES

This exercise focuses on the muscle on the middle of the shoulder, a relatively small muscle that supports many movements that we perform.

THE MOVEMENT

Stand with your arms hanging down at your sides and a dumbbell in each hand. Raise the dumbbells straight out to your sides until you're holding them at eye level, keeping your palms facing downward, and then lower them back down. This constitutes 1 rep.

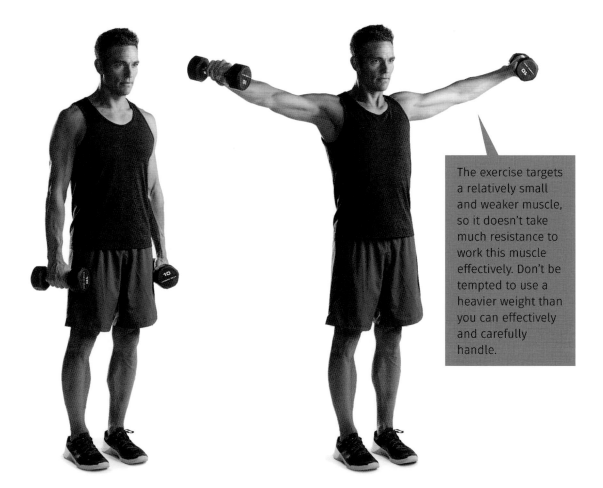

The exercise targets a relatively small and weaker muscle, so it doesn't take much resistance to work this muscle effectively. Don't be tempted to use a heavier weight than you can effectively and carefully handle.

PRIMARY MUSCLES WORKED

▶ Medial deltoids

SECONDARY MUSCLES WORKED

▶ Anterior deltoids
▶ Posterior deltoids
▶ Triceps
▶ Transverse abdominis

◀ LEVEL **1**

Perform **THE MOVEMENT** as described.

LEVEL **2**

Perform this exercise alternating one arm at a time. This destabilizes your body laterally as your center of gravity shifts outward toward the moving dumbbell, and so creates a greater challenge for your transverse abdominis.

LEVEL **3** ▶

Perform this exercise standing on one foot only, or standing on the soft side of a BOSU. For an additional challenge, perform this standing on one foot with a dumbbell only in the hand you are raising (as shown).

FRONT RAISES

This exercise targets the muscles of the front of the shoulder.

Hold a light dumbbell in each hand and let your arms hang down at your sides. Raise one arm forward until it is straight out in front of you at eye level with the palm facing downward. Slowly lower the dumbbell, and then raise and lower the other arm in the same fashion. This constitutes 1 rep.

As you bring your arm (or arms) forward, be sure to keep the rest of your body still. Rocking back and forth creates momentum and thus reduces the amount of work that the muscle is responsible for. Engage your transverse abdominis by tightening your core, and bend your knees slightly to engage your leg muscles. This helps anchor the movement.

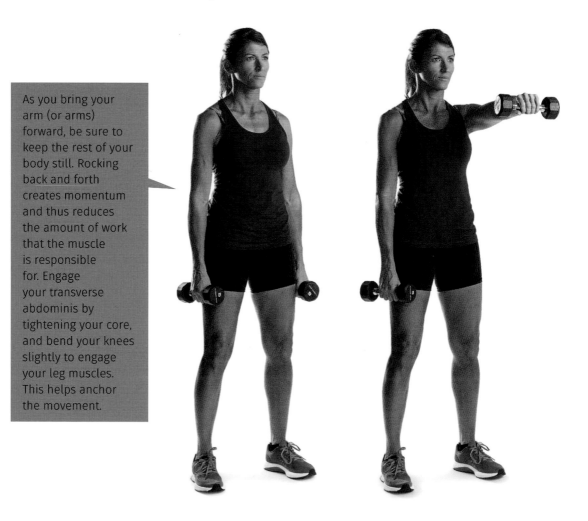

**PRIMARY
MUSCLES WORKED**

▶ Anterior deltoids

**SECONDARY
MUSCLES WORKED**

▶ Medial deltoids
▶ Posterior deltoids
▶ Transverse abdominis
▶ Erector spinae
▶ Calf muscles
  (in advanced form)

◀ LEVEL **1**

Perform **THE MOVEMENT** as
described. To raise the difficulty
level, try raising both arms
simultaneously. This shifts your
center of gravity forward a bit,
which increases the challenge to
your lower back to keep you from
falling forward.

LEVEL **2** ▶

Perform the exercise while
standing on one leg for half of
your repetitions, alternating
arms, and on the other leg for the
remainder of your set. For a more
difficult variation, raise both arms
at the same time (as shown).

LEVEL **3**

Perform this exercise while
standing on the soft side of a
BOSU. For a very challenging
alternative, try standing with
only one foot on the BOSU.

HIGH REVERSE FLYES

This exercise completes the trio of shoulder movements that target each of the muscles of the deltoid group. It targets the muscles of the rear shoulder, the most powerful of the three. By including a rotation movement, it also engages the muscles underneath the deltoid.

THE MOVEMENT

Stand with feet shoulder-width apart and hands close together near your lower waist. Keep your elbows bent and your palms facing your body. Swing your arms simultaneously up and away from your body until you are holding your arms wide just above eye level. Slowly let your arms swing back down, following the same arcing path that they took going up. This constitutes 1 rep.

Keep your body still while you're doing this exercise; you should not be rocking back and forth as your arms swing up and down. Bend forward slightly at the waist, and keep your knees slightly bent as well. This will help you control your foundation as your arms move your center of gravity around.

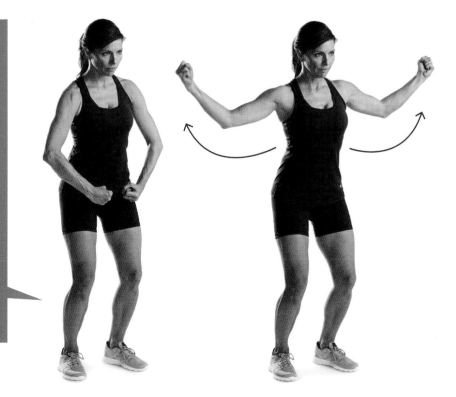

PRIMARY MUSCLES WORKED

▶ **Posterior deltoids**
▶ **Rear rotator cuff**

◀ LEVEL **1**

Perform **THE MOVEMENT** as described.

LEVEL **2**

Perform the exercise as described, adding light dumbbells.

SECONDARY MUSCLES WORKED

▶ **Biceps**
▶ **Transverse abdominis**

LEVEL **3** ▶

Perform this exercise as described in Level 2, while alternatively standing on one foot and then the other, or while standing on the soft side of a BOSU (as shown). You can move both arms simultaneously or increase the difficulty by alternating your arm swings.

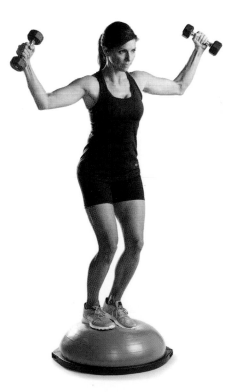

LOW REVERSE FLYES

This exercise targets the muscles of the middle upper back, between the shoulder blades. These muscles not only stabilize the movement of your arms, they also help maintain proper posture.

THE MOVEMENT

Stand with one foot in front of the other, holding a dumbbell in each hand. Bend over, about 10 degrees or so, and bend your knees slightly. The dumbbells should be touching out in front of you. Spread your arms wide, bringing your elbows back, as if trying to touch your elbows together behind your back. Return to the starting position by bringing your arms back together in front of you. This constitutes 1 rep.

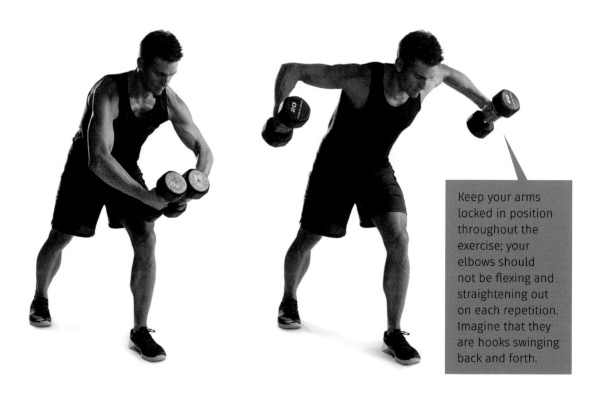

Keep your arms locked in position throughout the exercise; your elbows should not be flexing and straightening out on each repetition. Imagine that they are hooks swinging back and forth.

PRIMARY
MUSCLES WORKED

▶ Rhomboids

SECONDARY MUSCLES
WORKED

▶ Erector spinae
▶ Triceps
▶ Posterior deltoids

◀ LEVEL **1**

Perform **THE MOVEMENT** as described.

LEVEL **2**

Perform the exercise standing on one leg for half of your target repetitions and on the other leg for the remainder of your set.

LEVEL **3** ▶

Perform this exercise while standing atop the soft side of a BOSU (as shown). Feet should be side by side, rather than scissored, due to the limited surface space.

Keep your arms perpendicular to your body. Since you'll be bending over slightly, your hands should be pointing toward the floor in front of you a little bit, not pointing at your feet, which would put them too close to your body.

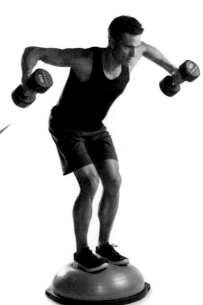

STANDING SHOULDER PRESSES

A shoulder press is a standard exercise for improving deltoid strength. Performing it from a standing position challenges the core to stabilize the body as weight moves farther from the body's center.

THE MOVEMENT

Standing a bit wider than shoulder width, hold a dumbbell in each hand, elbows bent, with forearms perpendicular to the ground. Looking toward the ceiling, raise the dumbbells up until your arms are almost straight and the dumbbells are touching overhead, then lower them. This constitutes 1 rep.

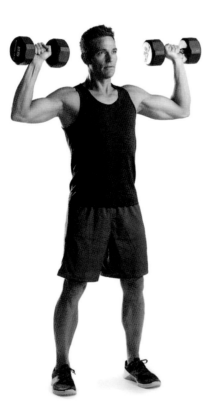

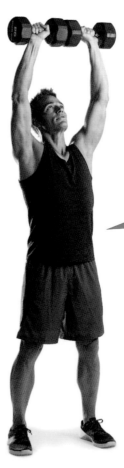

You will naturally arch your back while performing this exercise, but avoid arching too much, as this puts unnecessary pressure on the lower back.

▸ Deltoids
▸ Triceps

▸ **Transverse abdominis**

◂ LEVEL **1**

Perform **THE MOVEMENT** as described. To increase
the difficulty, perform the movement with one
dumbbell in one hand at a time. This puts more
stress on one side of the body than the other,
which creates lateral instability and forces the
core to work harder to stay in alignment.

LEVEL **2** ▸

Stand on one leg for half of the set, switching
to the other leg for the remaining repetitions.
Hold your dumbbell in the hand opposite to
your upraised foot, so that you remain more
balanced. Or, to up the challenge, perform the
press with the dumbbell held on the same side
as the upraised foot (as shown). This increases
the challenge on the unsupported side of your
body, which requires more core engagement.

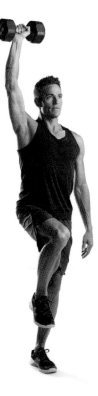

LEVEL **3**

Increase complexity by combining the shoulder
press with a squat. Holding the dumbbells at
shoulder level, squat and then stand up while
performing the shoulder press simultaneously.
This constitutes 1 rep.

MONKEY SQUATS

To get the most out of this exercise, you need to use a significant amount of weight, so this is a great one to do if you have access to a heavy dumbbell. The weight you use should feel challenging, but not oppressively so. Remember that you'll be working the largest, strongest muscles of the body, so don't underestimate your power. In fact, many people find that the greatest challenge of this exercise may not be to the legs but to the hands, which have to hold the weight.

THE MOVEMENT

Stand with feet shoulder-width apart and a heavy dumbbell positioned vertically on the floor directly below you. Squat, letting your arms hang down as a monkey might do. Grip the dumbbell with both hands on the top part of the weight. Keeping your pelvis tilted and your back arched, stand up until your knees are almost—but not quite—locked out. Then bend your knees and return to the starting position. This constitutes 1 rep.

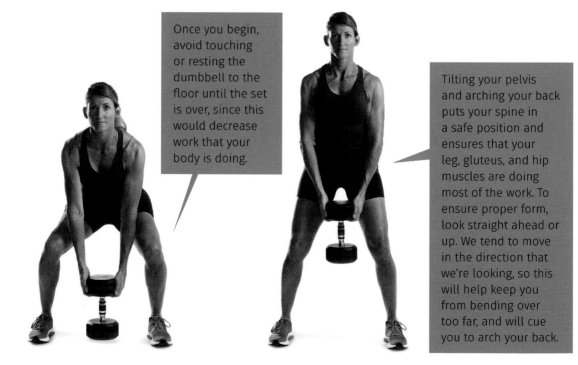

Once you begin, avoid touching or resting the dumbbell to the floor until the set is over, since this would decrease work that your body is doing.

Tilting your pelvis and arching your back puts your spine in a safe position and ensures that your leg, gluteus, and hip muscles are doing most of the work. To ensure proper form, look straight ahead or up. We tend to move in the direction that we're looking, so this will help keep you from bending over too far, and will cue you to arch your back.

PRIMARY MUSCLES WORKED

▸ Quadriceps
▸ Gluteus maximus
▸ Hamstrings

SECONDARY MUSCLES WORKED

▸ Erector spinae
▸ Gluteus medius
▸ Forearm flexors

LEVEL **1**

Perform the exercise as described but without a dumbbell.

◂ ## LEVEL **2**

Perform **THE MOVEMENT** as described.

LEVEL **3** ▸

Perform the exercise from atop the hard side of a BOSU (as shown). This increases the challenge by destabilizing your base, which requires your brain to figure out how to use your neuromuscular system to reestablish balance.

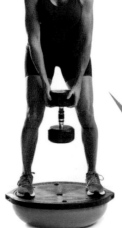

As you perform this exercise, imagine that your arms are cables running from your shoulders to the dumbbell. They are just hanging there. You should not engage the biceps by bending the elbows, since that limits the amount of weight that you can handle and reduces the challenge to the big muscles of your legs, hips, and backside.

ROLL OUTS

This exercise makes use of the ab wheel. It essentially requires you to perform a bridge, but it pushes that position farther, challenging the arms and shoulders, and also engaging the core through a range of motion. Along the way, it also forces the body to engage its lateral stabilizers.

THE MOVEMENT

Start on all fours, with your hands on the ab wheel's handles. Roll out until the wheel is just past your head, then return. That's 1 rep. It can take a few repetitions to loosen up, so don't expect that the range on your first repetition is as far as you can go.

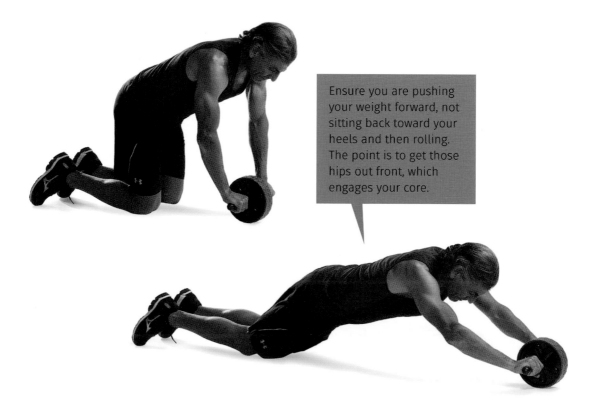

Ensure you are pushing your weight forward, not sitting back toward your heels and then rolling. The point is to get those hips out front, which engages your core.

▸ **Rectus abdominis**
▸ **Hip flexors**

LEVEL **1**

Perform **THE MOVEMENT** as described.

LEVEL **2**

Roll out until your nose is almost touching the floor, then return.

▸ **Erector spinae**
▸ **Deltoids**
▸ **Triceps**
▸ **Transverse abdominis**

LEVEL **3** ▸

Roll out as in Level 2, but keep your toes off the ground as you perform the exercise (as shown). Without the aid of your toes as an anchor, your core is forced to work harder.

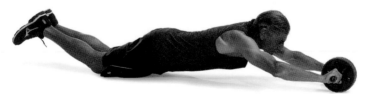

ROLL UPS

This is like a sit-up, but more challenging because you have less leverage than in a regular sit-up.

THE MOVEMENT

Lie flat on the floor with knees slightly bent and arms straight at your sides. Rise up into a sitting position while keeping your heels on the floor, then return to your starting position. That's 1 rep.

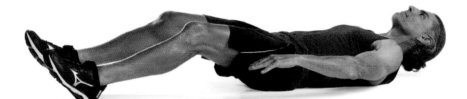

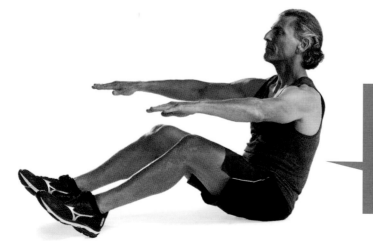

Don't fall backward too quickly; keep your abs engaged by lying back down slowly. Ensure that your heels stay on the floor throughout the movement.

PRIMARY MUSCLES WORKED

▸ Rectus abdominis
▸ Hip flexors

SECONDARY MUSCLES WORKED

▸ Erector spinae

◀ LEVEL **1**

Perform **THE MOVEMENT** as described.

LEVEL **2**

Perform the exercise as described above, but with legs extended rather than bent.

LEVEL **3** ▸

Keep your arms crossed over your chest throughout the movement (as shown). This prevents you from using your arms to create momentum on the way up, which puts more pressure on your abs.

HIP THRUSTS

This exercise works the core, backside, and hips, but it also challenges the arms, shoulders, and lower back by using these muscles to hold the reverse bridge position. With all of these muscles working, it's no surprise that this exercise might be harder than it looks.

THE MOVEMENT

Starting in a sitting position, put your palms on the floor behind you and rise up so that only your palms and heels are touching the floor. Keeping knees slightly bent, raise your hips up as far as possible and then lower them back down. Do not touch the ground; your body should be in the air throughout the exercise.

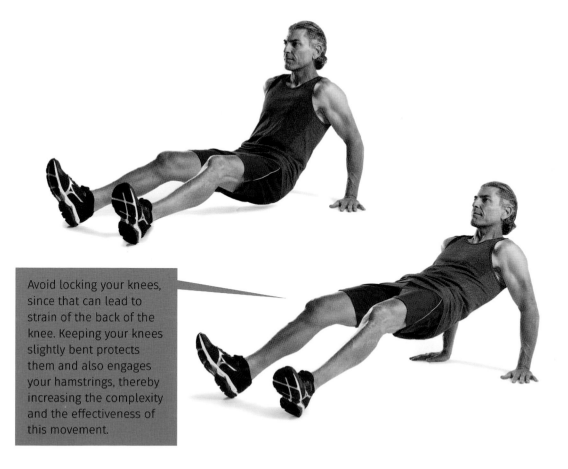

Avoid locking your knees, since that can lead to strain of the back of the knee. Keeping your knees slightly bent protects them and also engages your hamstrings, thereby increasing the complexity and the effectiveness of this movement.

▶ Gluteus maximus
▶ Gluteus medius
▶ Erector spinae

LEVEL **1**

Do the exercise as described, but start with your elbows and forearms on the floor, with knees bent and feet flat on the floor.

▶ Rectus abdominis
▶ Deltoids
▶ Triceps
▶ Hamstrings

◀ LEVEL **2**

Perform **THE MOVEMENT** as described. This exercise relies on extension of the shoulder, which can be difficult if you have a history of shoulder problems, so be on the lookout for shoulder pain. If you experience any discomfort or pain, drop down to the Level 1 movement.

LEVEL **3** ▶

Place your BOSU soft side up, and put your heels on top of it (as shown). Performing this exercise with a soft foundation for your heels challenges your core to work harder to stabilize your body.

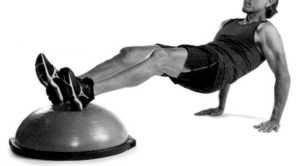

PUSH-UPS

This is the granddaddy of floor exercises, the one that we all remember from high school gym class. It is a highly effective strength builder, and a great test of your strength-to-body-weight ratio, as well as your overall fitness. That's because it tests your ability to keep your body straight and to hold it steady in space as you work your upper body. For this reason, I consider it a superior exercise to the bench press, which can present a greater challenge to your upper body but which doesn't significantly engage your core.

THE MOVEMENT

Lie facedown on the floor with your palms down on the floor next to you, just below shoulder height. Turn your hands inward slightly, so that your elbows point outward as well. Rise into a plank from your toes, and then bend your elbows and lower your body back down to the floor as far as you can without touching the ground. This constitutes 1 rep.

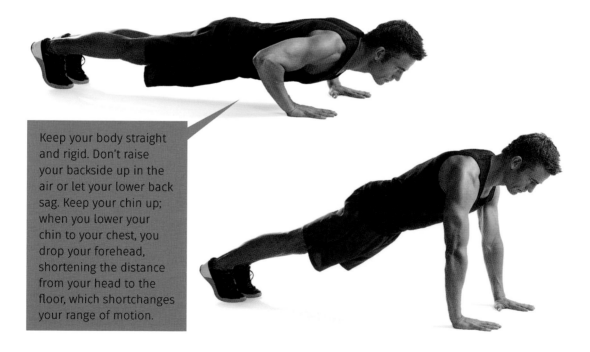

Keep your body straight and rigid. Don't raise your backside up in the air or let your lower back sag. Keep your chin up; when you lower your chin to your chest, you drop your forehead, shortening the distance from your head to the floor, which shortchanges your range of motion.

PRIMARY MUSCLES WORKED

▶ Chest
▶ Anterior deltoids
▶ Triceps

SECONDARY MUSCLES WORKED

▶ Rectus abdominis
▶ Gluteus maximus
▶ Erector spinae

LEVEL **1**

If you don't feel strong enough to perform this exercise from your toes, drop to your knees and do push-ups from there. Keep your body rigidly straight from your knees to your shoulders.

◀ LEVEL **2**

Perform **THE MOVEMENT** as described.

LEVEL **3** ▶

Raise one leg straight up behind you for half the set, and then raise the other leg for the remainder (as shown). This engages the gluteus maximus muscles and requires your body to balance itself a bit more.

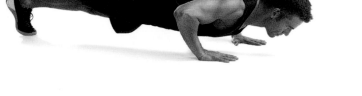

CRUNCHES

This exercise develops our "six-pack" muscles. Although it does not work the all-important transverse abdominis, other important abdominal muscles are engaged. This exercise also productively fills the gap between exercises as you wait for other muscle groups to recover.

THE MOVEMENT

Lie on your back with knees bent and hands held lightly behind your head or folded across your chest. Roll your shoulders up until your shoulder blades are off the floor, then return to the starting position. This constitutes 1 rep.

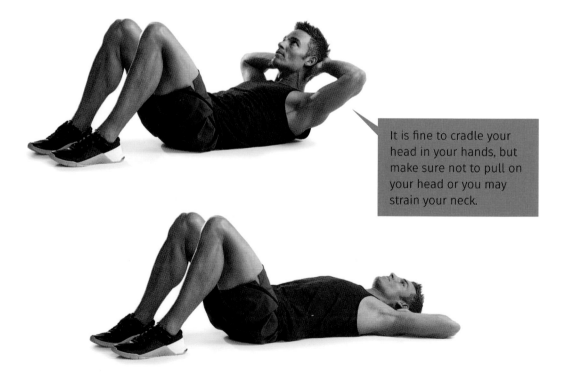

It is fine to cradle your head in your hands, but make sure not to pull on your head or you may strain your neck.

PRIMARY
MUSCLES WORKED

▶ Rectus abdominis

SECONDARY
MUSCLES WORKED

▶ Hip flexors
▶ Adductors (in advanced form)
▶ Quadriceps (in advanced form)

◀ LEVEL **1**

Perform **THE MOVEMENT** as described.

LEVEL **2**

Straighten your legs. This gives you less leverage, making this exercise more challenging.

LEVEL **3** ▶

Hold the stability ball between your ankles and keep it in the air as you perform this exercise (as shown). This engages the adductor muscles of your inner thighs, as well as your hip flexors and quadriceps muscles. For an even greater challenge, raise the ball up and down as you do the crunches.

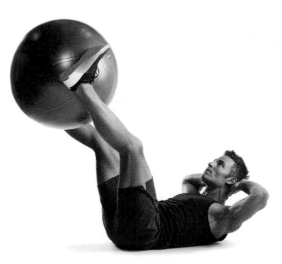

CROSSOVER CRUNCHES

This exercise focuses on rotation, which engages the side muscles. It provides a nice counterpoint to many of the other floor core exercises, which tend to move along the same plane, going up and down or forward and backward.

THE MOVEMENT

Lie faceup with your knees bent. Cross your left ankle over your right knee. Keeping your left arm on the floor and your right hand on the back of your head, bring your right shoulder up and across diagonally toward your left knee, and then return to the starting position. This constitutes 1 rep.

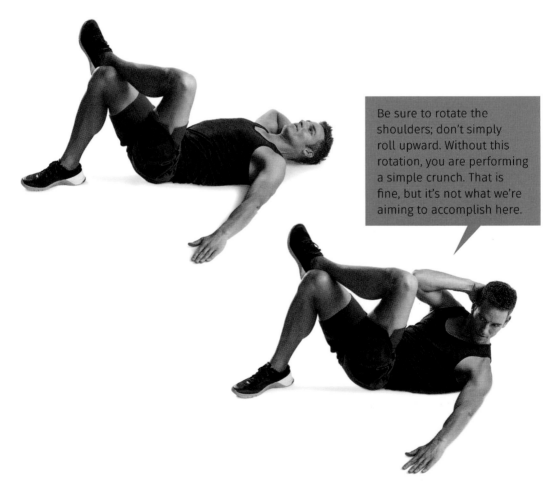

Be sure to rotate the shoulders; don't simply roll upward. Without this rotation, you are performing a simple crunch. That is fine, but it's not what we're aiming to accomplish here.

PRIMARY
MUSCLES WORKED

▶ Rectus abdominis
▶ Obliques

SECONDARY
MUSCLES WORKED

▶ Hip flexors
▶ Erector spinae

◀ LEVEL **1**

Perform **THE MOVEMENT** as described.

LEVEL **2**

Instead of placing your left ankle on your right knee, raise the left leg straight above you. The right knee remains bent, with that foot on the floor. As you begin your crossover crunch, raise the straightened leg and reach for it with the opposite arm as you extend that arm diagonally across your body. Aim to touch your elbow to the opposite knee. It doesn't matter if you actually do; the point is to engage the target muscle groups, which you can do without making contact with each repetition. Your knee is simply a target to aim for.

LEVEL **3** ▶

Perform the Level 2 crossover crunch on a BOSU. Place the palm of your opposite hand on the floor beside you as an anchor (as shown). As you become more comfortable with the instability of the BOSU, place this hand on your stomach.

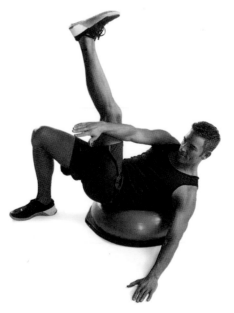

LEG RAISES

This is a single joint movement, involving just your hips, but it challenges many core muscles.

THE MOVEMENT

Lie faceup with your hands on the floor by your hips. You can place the edges of your hands under your backside to gain some stability, if necessary. Keep your knees extended and your legs together and straight. Raise your legs off the floor until they are perpendicular to the ground, then slowly lower them down again. This constitutes 1 rep.

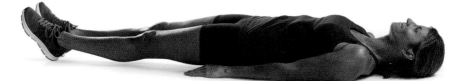

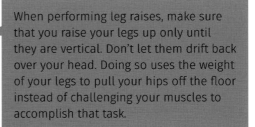

When performing leg raises, make sure that you raise your legs up only until they are vertical. Don't let them drift back over your head. Doing so uses the weight of your legs to pull your hips off the floor instead of challenging your muscles to accomplish that task.

PRIMARY MUSCLES WORKED

▶ Rectus abdominis
▶ Hip flexors

SECONDARY MUSCLES WORKED

▶ Erector spinae
▶ Transverse abdominis

◀ ### LEVEL **1**

Perform **THE MOVEMENT** as described. If this feels too difficult to perform with legs straight, bend your knees to gain leverage. As you feel stronger, straighten your legs out bit by bit.

LEVEL **2**

Squeeze a stability ball between your ankles and raise it up as you perform this exercise. This engages your adductor muscles. For a different challenge, instead of using your hands as an anchor, fold your hands over your belly, keeping elbows off the floor. This challenges your core to hold your body in place as your moving legs tug at your upper body.

For an additional challenge, with or without a stability ball, try not to touch the floor between repetitions when you return to the starting position.

LEVEL **3** ▶

Place your arms at your sides, with palms down on the floor. After you raise your legs up, push down against your palms and raise your hips off the floor (as shown). Then lower your hips back down, and lower your legs back down. Imagine that your legs are being pulled up towards the ceiling. Then lower your hips back down, and lower your legs back down. This engages your lower back and provides a greater challenge to your abdominals.

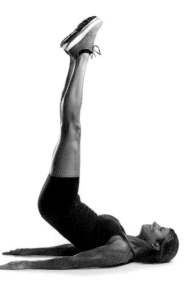

FIRE HYDRANTS

This exercise may feel a little silly, but rest assured that people all the world over do this simple, effective movement to strengthen their outer hips.

THE MOVEMENT

Begin on all fours. Raise your bent right leg out toward the side until it is parallel to the floor, and then lower it back down. This constitutes 1 rep.

Avoid rotating your body during this exercise, and aim to keep your hips parallel to the floor. If you rotate, you won't challenge your gluteus medius as much as you should. If you feel that you have limited range and can't get your leg parallel to the ground, go as far as you comfortably can and work on stretching.

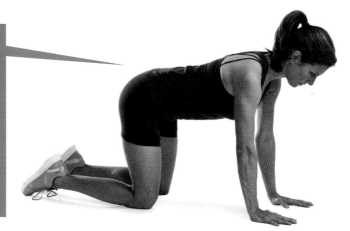

Be sure that your knee doesn't drift back as you raise your leg. Doing so will shift the focus to the gluteus maximus, which is not the muscle we're aiming to work on here. The thigh of your moving leg should remain perpendicular to your body throughout the movement.

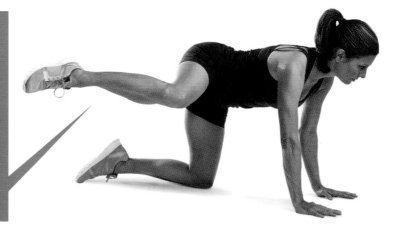

**PRIMARY
MUSCLES WORKED**

▶ Gluteus medius

**SECONDARY
MUSCLES WORKED**

▶ Transverse abdominis
▶ Chest
▶ Triceps

◀ LEVEL **1**

Perform **THE MOVEMENT** as described.

LEVEL **2** ▶

Perform this exercise from all fours atop the soft side of a BOSU (as shown).

LEVEL **3**

Perform as described in Level 1, but reach out and forward with the arm opposite your raised leg. This removes one of the supports for your body, which destabilizes you and challenges your core to keep you from toppling over. Add another challenge by keeping the toes of your supporting leg off the floor as well. This leaves you with just one hand and one knee touching the ground. Keep your balance by focusing on actively engaging your transverse abdominis.

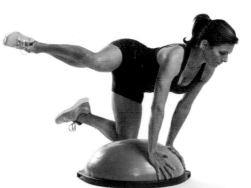

DONKEY KICKS

This exercise focuses on the powerful muscles of your backside.

THE MOVEMENT

Beginning on all fours, kick your right leg behind you, and then return to the starting position. You can perform this exercise by either keeping your knee bent while aiming to raise your heel up toward the ceiling (as shown) or by straightening your leg as you push back, as if you were kicking someone behind you. This constitutes 1 rep.

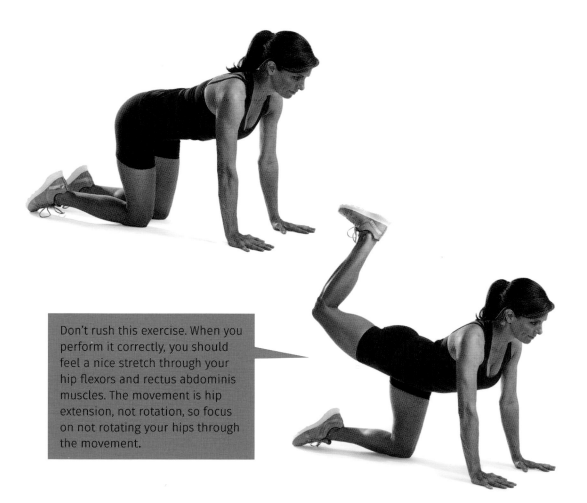

Don't rush this exercise. When you perform it correctly, you should feel a nice stretch through your hip flexors and rectus abdominis muscles. The movement is hip extension, not rotation, so focus on not rotating your hips through the movement.

**PRIMARY
MUSCLES WORKED**

▸ Gluteus maximus

**SECONDARY
MUSCLES WORKED**

▸ Transverse abdominis
▸ Chest
▸ Triceps

◀ LEVEL **1**

Perform **THE MOVEMENT** as described.

LEVEL **2**

Perform this exercise from atop the soft side of a BOSU.

LEVEL **3** ▶

Perform as described in Level 1, but raise the opposite arm off the floor. This removes one of the supports for your body, which destabilizes you, challenging your core to keep you from toppling over. To really up the difficulty, lift your toes off the ground as well so you are resting on one knee and one hand only (as shown).

SUPERMANS

This exercise works some of the strongest muscles in your body, and it will help keep your lower back strong and injury free.

THE MOVEMENT

Lie facedown with your arms outstretched in front of you. Arch your body upward, raising your shoulders and legs simultaneously, and then lower down. This constitutes 1 rep. If you have difficulty, focus on raising your arms and shoulders only. Bend your elbows and keep your arms closer to your body if necessary; this gives you more leverage and reduces the challenge of holding up your shoulders. Once you feel strong performing this movement, begin raising your legs and straightening your arms.

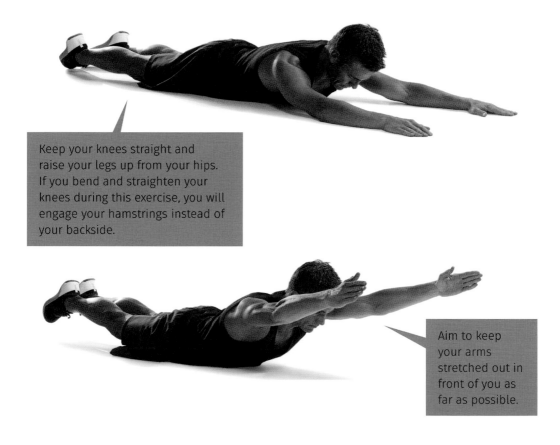

Keep your knees straight and raise your legs up from your hips. If you bend and straighten your knees during this exercise, you will engage your hamstrings instead of your backside.

Aim to keep your arms stretched out in front of you as far as possible.

PRIMARY MUSCLES WORKED

▶ Gluteus maximus
▶ Erector spinae

SECONDARY MUSCLES WORKED

▶ Posterior deltoids
▶ Latissimus dorsi
▶ Rhomboids

◀ LEVEL **1**

Perform **THE MOVEMENT** as described.

LEVEL **2** ▶

Perform this exercise atop the soft side of a BOSU (as shown). You might find yourself teeter-tottering at first, but once you find your balance point, it won't be hard to coordinate your movement. Use your arms to find that point.

LEVEL **3**

Hold a light pair of dumbbells out in front of you. This further challenges your rear deltoids.

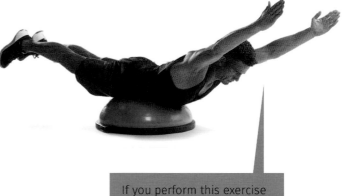

If you perform this exercise from atop a BOSU, you can use your arms to adjust your balance, similar to the way a high-wire walker uses a balance pole to regulate body position.

SIDE CRUNCHES

This exercise builds strength in some of your lateral stabilizers.

THE MOVEMENT

Lie on your left side, keeping your body as straight as possible. Simultaneously raise up your legs from your hips and your shoulders, and then lower both back down. This constitutes 1 rep.

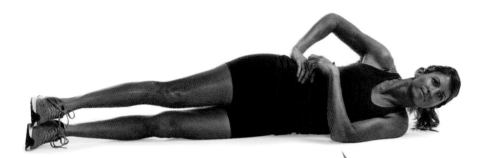

You can keep your lower arm tucked in alongside your body, but rely on that arm for balance only; do not push off with it, since this reduces the challenge on our target muscle group, the obliques. As for where to put your hands, I like to keep them on my upward-facing obliques, since this feels comfortable and also allows me to feel my obliques working, which assures me that I'm performing the exercise correctly.

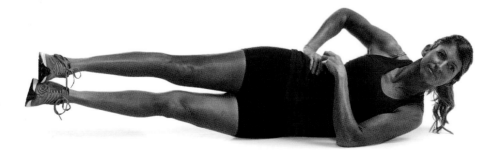

PRIMARY MUSCLES WORKED

▸ Obliques

SECONDARY MUSCLES WORKED

▸ Gluteus medius

LEVEL **1**

Rather than raising your upper body and your lower body simultaneously, which ups the level of difficulty, keep your upper body on the floor and focus on raising only your legs. If needed, put a small pillow or folded towel under your head.

◂ ## LEVEL **2**

Perform **THE MOVEMENT** as described. You can make it harder by not letting your legs or upper body touch the ground between repetitions. This prevents the working muscles from resting throughout the set.

LEVEL **3** ▸

Lie sideways on the soft side of your BOSU, placing your top hand on your hip and your lower hand either on the floor or on the BOSU for balance (as shown). Perform this exercise without letting your legs touch the ground.

SIDE LEG RAISES

This exercise can feel quite difficult, as it focuses on a single muscle group and requires that this muscle lift a relatively heavy load.

THE MOVEMENT

Lie on your right side with legs outstretched, knees extended, and left leg on top of the right. Place a small pillow or folded towel under your head to avoid neck strain. Keep your elbows tucked in at your sides. Raise the top leg as high as you comfortably can, and lower it back down again. This constitutes 1 rep.

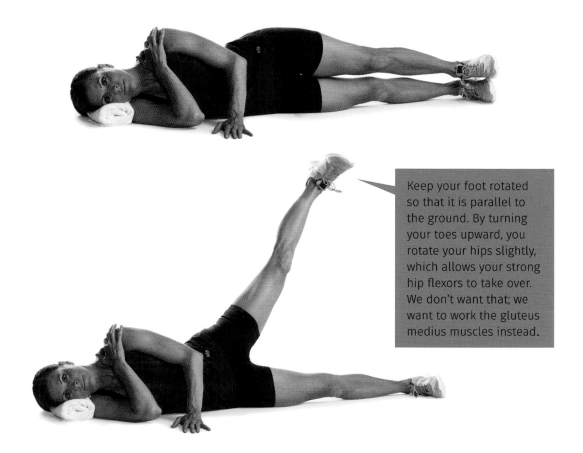

Keep your foot rotated so that it is parallel to the ground. By turning your toes upward, you rotate your hips slightly, which allows your strong hip flexors to take over. We don't want that; we want to work the gluteus medius muscles instead.

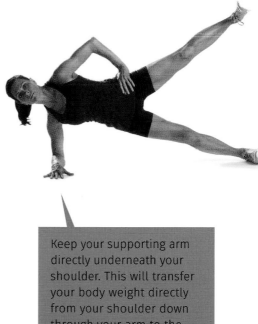

PRIMARY MUSCLES WORKED

▶ Gluteus medius

SECONDARY MUSCLES WORKED

▶ Gluteus maximus
▶ Obliques (in advanced forms)

◀ LEVEL **1**

Perform **THE MOVEMENT** as described, aiming to raise your leg up as high as possible.

LEVEL **2** ▶

Perform from a side plank position, balancing on one elbow with the palm of your top hand on your hip (as shown). This movement requires you to balance on one elbow and one foot, which engages your transverse abdominis. You also engage your oblique muscles, which are working hard to keep your body straight.

LEVEL **3**

Perform this exercise from a side plank position, as in Level 2, but hold your top arm straight up in the air. This moves some of your body weight away from your center, which makes keeping your balance harder. To increase the challenge, hold a light dumbbell in the raised hand. By moving the dumbbell to different positions—slightly in front or behind you—you can appreciate how a slight change in body position increases the challenge of this exercise.

Keep your supporting arm directly underneath your shoulder. This will transfer your body weight directly from your shoulder down through your arm to the floor. If your elbow strays out farther, it will put undue pressure on your shoulder.

PULLOVERS

This exercise challenges the shoulders and provides a good stretch across your back and rib cage.

THE MOVEMENT

Lie on your back with your knees slightly bent and heels on the floor. Hold a single dumbbell with both hands directly over your body, with your elbows slightly bent and your arms perpendicular to the floor. Start the movement with the dumbbell held perpendicular to the floor. While keeping your arms slightly bent, lower the dumbbell over your head toward the floor, and then raise it back up to a vertical position. This constitutes 1 rep.

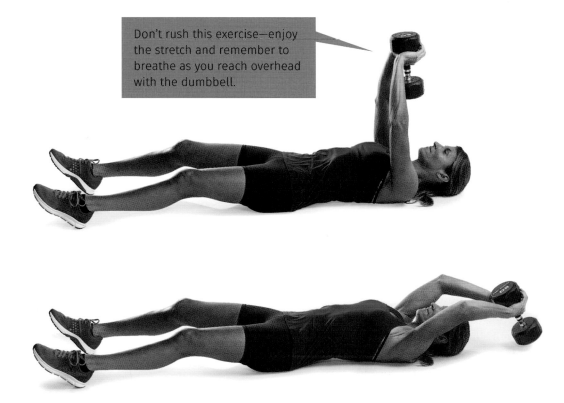

Don't rush this exercise—enjoy the stretch and remember to breathe as you reach overhead with the dumbbell.

PRIMARY MUSCLES WORKED

▶ Deltoids

SECONDARY MUSCLES WORKED

▶ Serratus anterior
▶ Triceps
▶ Erector spinae
▶ Transverse abdominis (in advanced form)
▶ Obliques (in advanced form)

◀ LEVEL **1**

Perform **THE MOVEMENT** as described. To raise the difficulty, do the exercise one arm at a time using a lighter dumbbell, performing all the repetitions with one hand and then switching to the other hand. This requires the shoulder to balance the weight laterally in addition to pulling it back and forth overhead.

LEVEL **2**

Increase the complexity by combining the pullover with leg raises. Keeping your legs straight, raise them up at the same time that you're pulling the dumbbell back to its vertical position, and then lower your legs as you lower the dumbbell to the floor over your head.

LEVEL **3** ▶

Perform this exercise while lying back on the soft side of a BOSU or from atop a stability ball with your head supported (as shown). This destabilizes your foundation, which challenges your transverse abdominis and obliques to maintain your balance during the exercise.

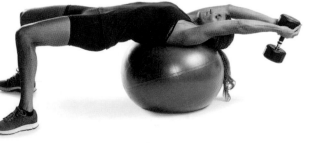

ADDUCTOR LEG RAISES

All movement requires the careful orchestration of muscle contractions by the body. Walking and running are particularly complex movements. Keeping the various muscle groups strong enough to complete their task will help avoid injury. The muscles of the inner thigh are one such group, and this exercise is designed to challenge them in an easy and efficient way.

THE MOVEMENT

Lie on your right side. Bend the knee of your left leg and place the left foot on the ground in front of the right knee. Your lower arm can be kept on the floor, and your upper arm may be kept on your upward-facing side. Keeping the right leg straight, raise it up as high as possible, and then lower it again. This constitutes 1 rep.

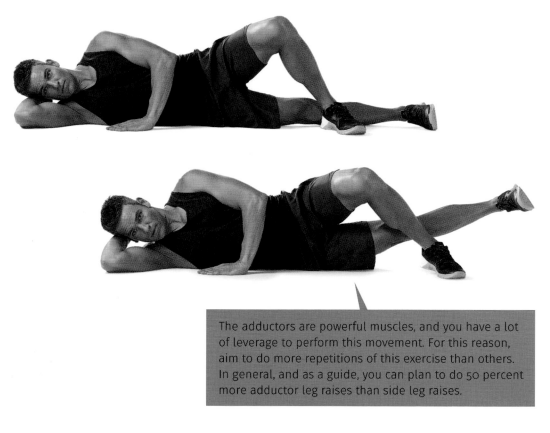

The adductors are powerful muscles, and you have a lot of leverage to perform this movement. For this reason, aim to do more repetitions of this exercise than others. In general, and as a guide, you can plan to do 50 percent more adductor leg raises than side leg raises.

PRIMARY MUSCLES WORKED

▶ Adductors

SECONDARY MUSCLES WORKED

▶ Hip flexors
▶ Obliques (in advanced form)
▶ Gluteus medius (in advanced form)

◀ LEVEL **1**

Perform **THE MOVEMENT** as described.

LEVEL **2**

Perform this exercise while holding a light dumbbell in the air.

LEVEL **3** ▶

Lying on your right side, rise to a side plank position, supported by your right elbow and the insole of your left foot, keeping the body as straight as possible. Supported by the left leg, with right leg slightly forward on the floor, raise and lower right leg (as shown). What makes this exercise so difficult is that in addition to the basic movement, you are now engaging your obliques and gluteus medius muscles in order to hold your body up in the air.

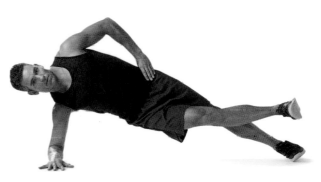

WINDSHIELD WIPERS

This rotation movement provides a good challenge to your core, and it also delivers a nice stretch to your outer hips.

THE MOVEMENT

Lie faceup, and hold your legs up in the air as straight as possible. Spread your arms out, perpendicular to your body, with palms down. Keeping your legs together, swing them down to your left side as far as you comfortably can, and then swing them in one smooth motion over to your right side. This constitutes 1 rep.

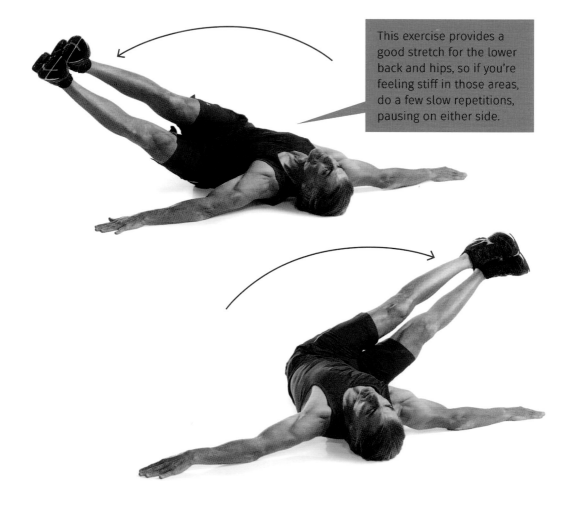

This exercise provides a good stretch for the lower back and hips, so if you're feeling stiff in those areas, do a few slow repetitions, pausing on either side.

PRIMARY MUSCLES WORKED

▶ Obliques

SECONDARY MUSCLES WORKED

▶ Hip flexors
▶ Rectus abdominis
▶ Erector spinae
▶ Adductors (in advanced form)

LEVEL 1

Perform the exercise as described, but with your knees bent. Physics teaches us that the shorter a lever is, the easier it is to move; bending your knees shortens that lever.

◀ LEVEL 2

Perform **THE MOVEMENT** as described.

LEVEL 3 ▶

Hold a stability ball between your ankles (as shown). This provides resistance to challenge your abdominals, and more importantly, it engages your adductor muscles as you squeeze your legs together to keep the ball from popping loose. Further challenge yourself by bringing your arms in closer to your sides.

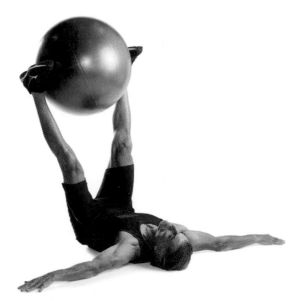

FUNCTIONAL

136 Mountain Climbers

138 Walking Lunges

140 Side Lunges

142 Step-Ups

144 Deadlift and Front Raises

146 Dumbbell Swings

148 Torso Twists

150 Lawn Mower Rows

152 Dumbbell Punches

154 Discus Throws

MOUNTAIN CLIMBERS

This exercise is tougher than it looks because you will work hard simply to hold the position even before you begin the movement. With so many muscle groups involved, this is a highly efficient and effective exercise.

THE MOVEMENT

Assume a basic plank position, as if you were about to perform a push-up. Draw your right knee up toward your right elbow, touching it if you can. Then push the knee back out again. Repeat with your left leg. This constitutes 1 rep.

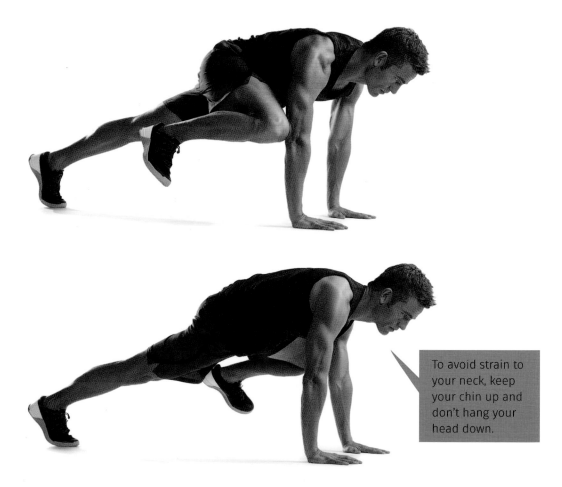

To avoid strain to your neck, keep your chin up and don't hang your head down.

PRIMARY MUSCLES WORKED

▶ Hip flexors

SECONDARY MUSCLES WORKED

▶ Chest
▶ Triceps
▶ Rectus abdominis

◀ ## LEVEL **1**

Perform **THE MOVEMENT** as described.

LEVEL **2** ▶

Increase the speed so that both legs are moving simultaneously, as though you are running in place (as shown).

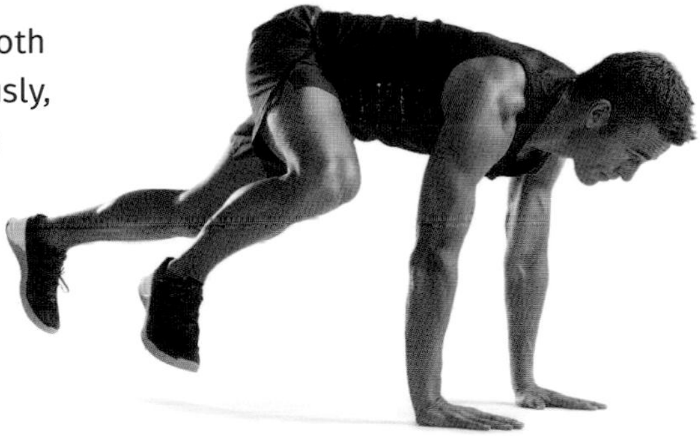

LEVEL **3**

Combine this exercise with push-ups to increase the challenge to your upper body.

WALKING LUNGES

This exercise requires your body to balance itself in space and then challenges it to recalibrate that balance as you move forward and continually change the position of your limbs.

THE MOVEMENT

Locate a stretch of floor that is at least 30 feet long. Keep your eyes focused on a distant point that's at about eye level, and hold your arms raised out to your sides. Take a long step forward with your right foot and sink downward, aiming to almost touch your back knee to the ground. Step forward with your left leg to meet your right, pausing slightly with your feet together, and then step forward with your left leg. This constitutes 1 rep.

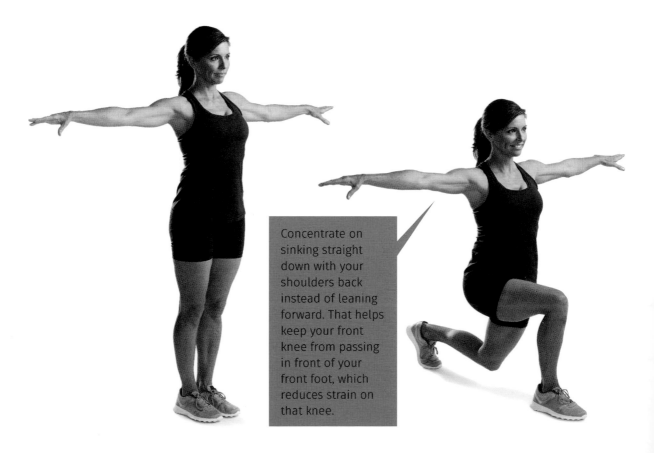

Concentrate on sinking straight down with your shoulders back instead of leaning forward. That helps keep your front knee from passing in front of your front foot, which reduces strain on that knee.

**PRIMARY
MUSCLES WORKED**

▶ Quadriceps
▶ Hamstrings
▶ Gluteus maximus
▶ Gluteus medius
▶ Anterior deltoids (in
advanced form)

**SECONDARY
MUSCLES WORKED**

▶ Gluteus medius
▶ Transverse abdominis

◀ LEVEL **1**

Perform **THE MOVEMENT** as described.

LEVEL **2**

Hold a dumbbell in front of you as you lunge, keeping your arms as straight as possible and your eyes on the dumbbell. This not only works your anterior deltoids but it also shifts your center of gravity forward. The weight challenges your lower back to work harder to keep you balanced and to combat falling forward.

LEVEL **3** ▶

For an even tougher challenge, try a walking lunge with a twist. Hold a lightweight dumbbell with both hands, and as you lunge forward, twist your upper body as you swing the dumbbell across your forward leg (as shown). Return to standing position, with feet together. Pause, and then swing the dumbbell to the other side as you continue lunging.

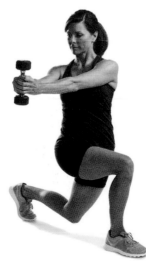

SIDE LUNGES

This exercise focuses on outer hip strength.

THE MOVEMENT

This exercise is similar to the standard squat but focuses more directly on the lateral stabilizers. Stand with your feet close together, knees slightly bent, and back slightly arched. Step out to the left, keeping your right leg straight as you bend your left knee down to a 90-degree angle. Step back up and lunge out to the right, keeping your left leg straight this time as you bend your right knee. This constitutes 1 rep.

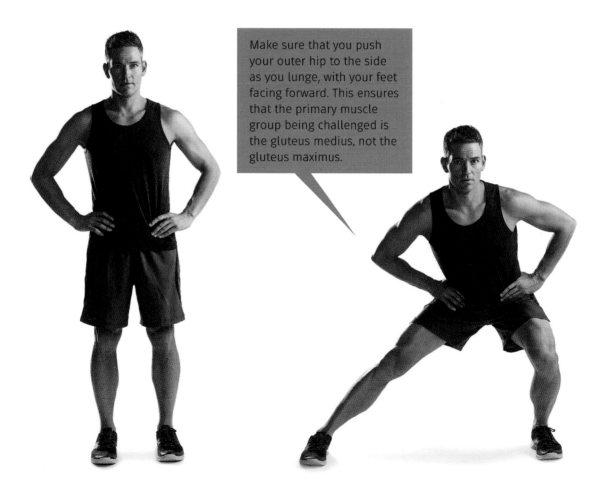

Make sure that you push your outer hip to the side as you lunge, with your feet facing forward. This ensures that the primary muscle group being challenged is the gluteus medius, not the gluteus maximus.

PRIMARY
MUSCLES WORKED

▸ Gluteus medius
▸ Quadriceps
▸ Hamstrings

◀ LEVEL **1**

Perform **THE MOVEMENT** as described.

SECONDARY
MUSCLES WORKED

▸ Transverse abdominis
▸ Erector spinae

LEVEL **2**

Focus on going lower and slower with each repetition.

LEVEL **3** ▶

Hold a light dumbbell or medicine ball straight out in front of you (as shown). This shifts your center of gravity forward slightly, putting more pressure on your lower back to keep you from pitching forward, thereby engaging those muscles to a greater degree.

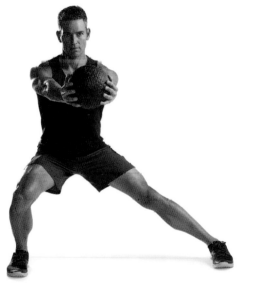

STEP-UPS

This exercise is a popular running drill in which a specific movement in the running motion is emphasized in order to build strength and coordination for running. The value of this exercise transcends running, however, since it incorporates a complex movement that engages several muscle groups while challenging your ability to keep your balance, so non-runners should include this exercise in their training.

THE MOVEMENT

Stand with your elbows bent, holding your left arm and right leg forward and your right arm and left leg back—basically, opposite arms and legs. Swing your right arm forward as you swing up your left knee. Reverse to return to the starting position. This is 1 rep.

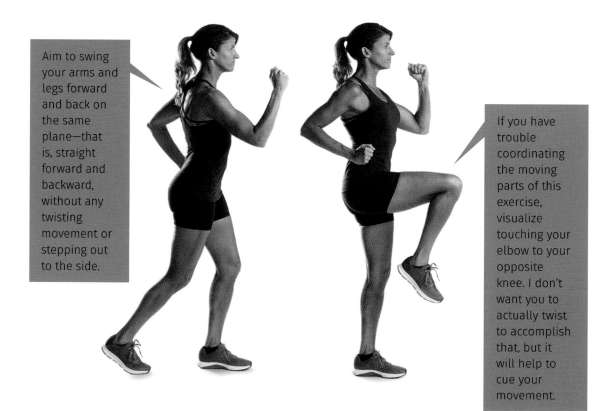

Aim to swing your arms and legs forward and back on the same plane—that is, straight forward and backward, without any twisting movement or stepping out to the side.

If you have trouble coordinating the moving parts of this exercise, visualize touching your elbow to your opposite knee. I don't want you to actually twist to accomplish that, but it will help to cue your movement.

**PRIMARY
MUSCLES WORKED**

▸ Hip flexors
▸ Gastrocnemius and soleus

◄ LEVEL **1**

Perform **THE MOVEMENT** as described.

LEVEL **2** ▸

Squat and bend your knees even more during this movement (as shown). This motion engages your legs even more by incorporating a squat or lunge motion in the exercise.

**SECONDARY
MUSCLES WORKED**

▸ Deltoids
▸ Transverse abdominis

LEVEL **3**

Perform this exercise with more intensity, letting the force of your raised knee lift you up onto your toes at the apex of each repetition. Another way to increase the difficulty is to start with your planted foot on a step or stair, forcing you to elevate even higher as you go through the motion. Alternatively, hold a medicine ball with arms straight out while you perform the lunge.

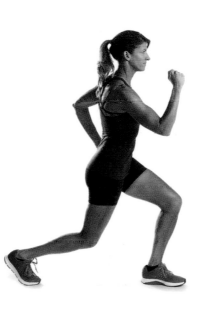

DEADLIFT AND FRONT RAISES

This exercise combines two simple movements into a single exercise that is greater than the sum of its parts.

THE MOVEMENT

Take a stance a bit wider than shoulder width. Bend forward from the hips, back arched, knees slightly bent, and grip a medium-weight dumbbell or medicine ball with both hands. Straighten up and swing the weight over your head toward the ceiling in one smooth movement. Hold it for just a moment, and then swing the weight back down. This constitutes 1 rep.

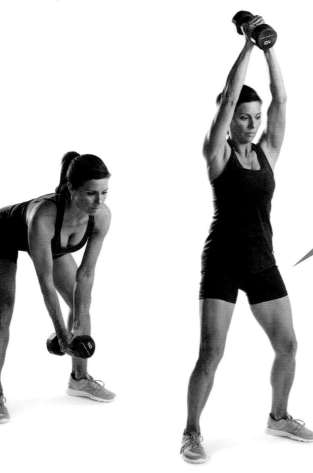

Make sure that you engage your hips rather than your mid-back by tilting your pelvis backward and arching your back. Ensure your knees stay in a slightly bent position.

PRIMARY MUSCLES WORKED

▶ Erector spinae
▶ Rear deltoids

SECONDARY MUSCLES WORKED

▶ Transverse abdominis
▶ Gluteus maximus

◀ LEVEL **1**

Perform **THE MOVEMENT** as described.

LEVEL **2**

Increase the intensity by making the movement ballistic. Do this by swinging the weight quickly and coming to a hard stop at the top and bottom of the movement. The hard stop increases the challenge to your core muscles as they engage to stop the momentum. Note: This version presents a higher risk of injury than the Level 1 version, especially if you don't use proper form, so be cautious and careful when performing this exercise.

LEVEL **3** ▶

Perform this movement while standing on the soft side of a BOSU. For a tougher challenge, flip the BOSU and stand on the hard side (as shown).

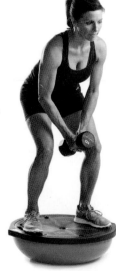

DUMBBELL SWINGS

This complex movement is highly functional, engaging your muscles in a movement pattern that's similar to the way you would accomplish a number of real-life tasks, such as shoveling snow.

THE MOVEMENT

Stand with feet shoulder-width apart, knees slightly bent. Hold a dumbbell with both hands against your outer hip. Keeping your arms as straight as possible, swing the weight up and out diagonally toward your other side until the weight is a little higher than eye level, and then return to the starting position. This constitutes 1 rep.

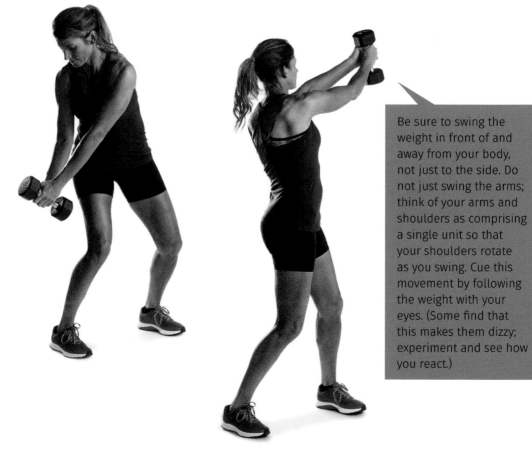

Be sure to swing the weight in front of and away from your body, not just to the side. Do not just swing the arms; think of your arms and shoulders as comprising a single unit so that your shoulders rotate as you swing. Cue this movement by following the weight with your eyes. (Some find that this makes them dizzy; experiment and see how you react.)

PRIMARY
MUSCLES WORKED

- Obliques
- Deltoids
- Erector spinae

SECONDARY
MUSCLES WORKED

- Transverse abdominis
- Rhomboids
- Latissimus dorsi
- Biceps
- Triceps

◀ LEVEL **1**

Perform **THE MOVEMENT** as described.

LEVEL **2** ▶

Perform this exercise with your feet together (as shown), which decreases stability and further engages your lateral stabilizing muscles, including your gluteus medius, abductors, and adductors.

Engage your legs by bending your knees even more on the downswing and straightening them on the upswing. This will introduce a modified squat movement, which further engages your legs and hips.

LEVEL **3**

Perform this exercise from atop the soft side of a BOSU.

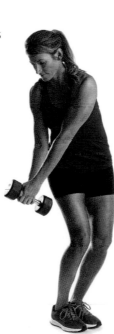

TORSO TWISTS

This rotation exercise builds strength very effectively for the sides and core.

Stand with feet shoulder-width apart. Hold a medium-weight dumbbell straight out in front of you with both hands. Keeping arms slightly bent, swing the dumbbell evenly from right to left and back again, on a trajectory parallel to the floor. This constitutes 1 rep.

Follow the dumbbell with your eyes throughout the movement. This cues your body to rotate more and helps you avoid simply swinging your arms instead of twisting. Some people find this makes them dizzy. If that's the case for you, avoid turning your head and focus instead on making sure that your body is moving correctly.

PRIMARY
MUSCLES WORKED

▸ Obliques

SECONDARY
MUSCLES WORKED

▸ Transverse abdominis
▸ Front deltoids

◀ LEVEL **1**

Perform **THE MOVEMENT** as described.

LEVEL **2** ▶

Keep your feet closer together—touching, even (as shown). This reduces your ability to distribute your weight across both feet, which in turn reduces your stability and challenges you to work harder to balance.

LEVEL **3**

Make the exercise ballistic by swinging the dumbbell faster, with a hard stop on either side. The hard stop directly engages your obliques in a very apparent way.

LAWN MOWER ROWS

This is a variation on a standard exercise, changed to make it an effective core strength builder.

THE MOVEMENT

Hold a dumbbell in your right hand, arm extended downward, with the right leg back and the left leg positioned forward. Bending forward slightly from the waist, pull the dumbbell upward to your armpit, swinging the other arm in the opposite direction, and then lower it down again. This constitutes 1 rep.

Keep in mind that this is mainly a torso rotation exercise. The unweighted arm is moving in order to help cue you to rotate your shoulders. This rotation mostly powers the movement of the dumbbell. If you're doing most of the work with your arm, you're not performing this exercise in the most effective way.

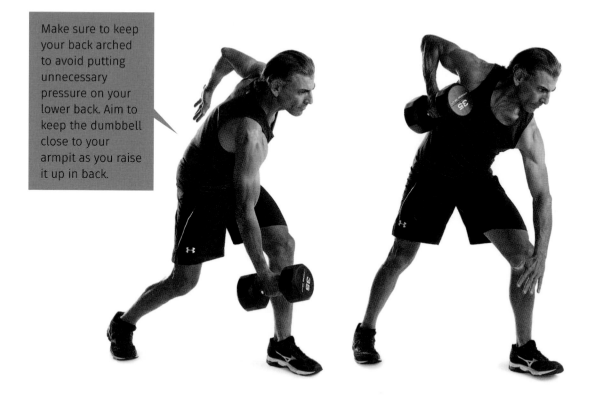

Make sure to keep your back arched to avoid putting unnecessary pressure on your lower back. Aim to keep the dumbbell close to your armpit as you raise it up in back.

PRIMARY MUSCLES WORKED

- ▶ Latissimus dorsi
- ▶ Posterior deltoids
- ▶ Obliques
- ▶ Biceps

SECONDARY MUSCLES WORKED

- ▶ Transverse abdominis

◀ LEVEL **1**

Perform **THE MOVEMENT** as directed.

LEVEL **2**

Perform the exercise with your eyes closed. This will feel disorienting at first, but you will soon get the hang of it.

LEVEL **3** ▶

Begin the exercise with your knees deeply bent (as shown), and then straighten them as your pull the dumbbell upward. This adds a squat to the exercise, further engaging the leg and hips.

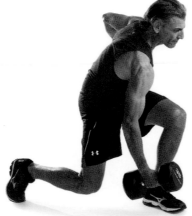

DUMBBELL PUNCHES

This exercise effectively combines rotation with a chest and shoulder exercise.

THE MOVEMENT

Assume a fighting position, with your left foot and left shoulder forward, right foot and right shoulder back. Your feet should be about a foot apart, with your left foot pointing forward and the right foot slightly angled for balance. Keeping your back slightly rounded, cock your right elbow back, with your forearm parallel to the floor. Position your left arm forward, perpendicular to the floor, with your fist near your chin. Rotate your shoulders as you push your right arm forward. As your hips turn and you follow through with a punch, allow the right foot to rotate. After straightening your arm, rotate back as you draw your right arm back to its starting position. This constitutes 1 rep.

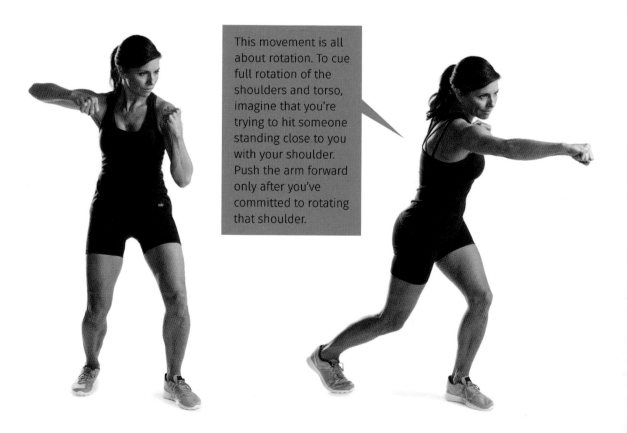

This movement is all about rotation. To cue full rotation of the shoulders and torso, imagine that you're trying to hit someone standing close to you with your shoulder. Push the arm forward only after you've committed to rotating that shoulder.

▸ Chest
▸ Anterior deltoids
▸ Triceps

▸ Transverse abdominis

◁ LEVEL **1**

Perform **THE MOVEMENT** as described.

LEVEL **2**

Perform this exercise as described, but holding a dumbbell in the punching hand.

LEVEL **3** ▶

Perform this exercise with a dumbbell in each hand (as shown). This puts an additional challenge on both shoulders, which will be engaged in keeping your now-heavier arms in position.

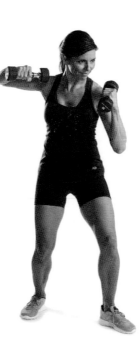

DISCUS THROWS

This complex exercise involves movement on many planes, working a wide range of muscle groups and challenging your balance as well. For these reasons, it might be one of the most efficient exercises you can do.

THE MOVEMENT

This exercise takes its name from the ancient Greek statue the Discobolus. But instead of holding a discus in your upraised arm, as the statue does, you hold a dumbbell in your lower hand.

   Place your left foot in front of you. Holding a dumbbell in your right hand, bend over slightly and squat, twisting as you descend, placing your right hand on the outside of your left knee, with the palm facing inward toward the knee. This is the starting position. In one smooth movement, stand up and rotate your body, toward your right. As you do so, swing your arm up and out, rotating it as you go. At the top of the movement, you should be standing up with your body rotated toward your right, with your right arm behind you. Return to the starting position by squatting and rotating toward your left, lowering your right arm back toward the outside of your left knee. This constitutes 1 rep.

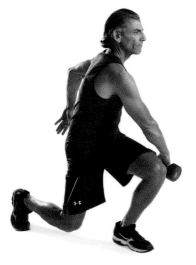

Keep in mind the image of a corkscrew as you perform this exercise. Instead of bending over as you descend, you should be turning and coming straight down. Similarly, you should be turning but not bending over as you stand up.

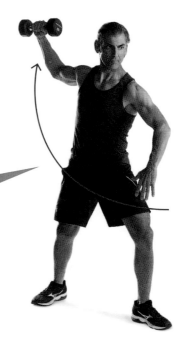

▸ Obliques
▸ Deltoids
▸ Gluteus maximus
▸ Quadriceps
▸ Hamstrings

▸ Transverse abdominis
▸ Gluteus medius

LEVEL **1**

Perform the exercise, but without a dumbbell. Focus simply on mastering the movement.

◀ ## LEVEL **2**

Perform **THE MOVEMENT** as described.

LEVEL **3** ▶

Perform the exercise while standing on one leg only (as shown). This requires you to pivot over the planted leg and rotate back around, which is a very challenging variation.

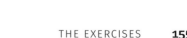

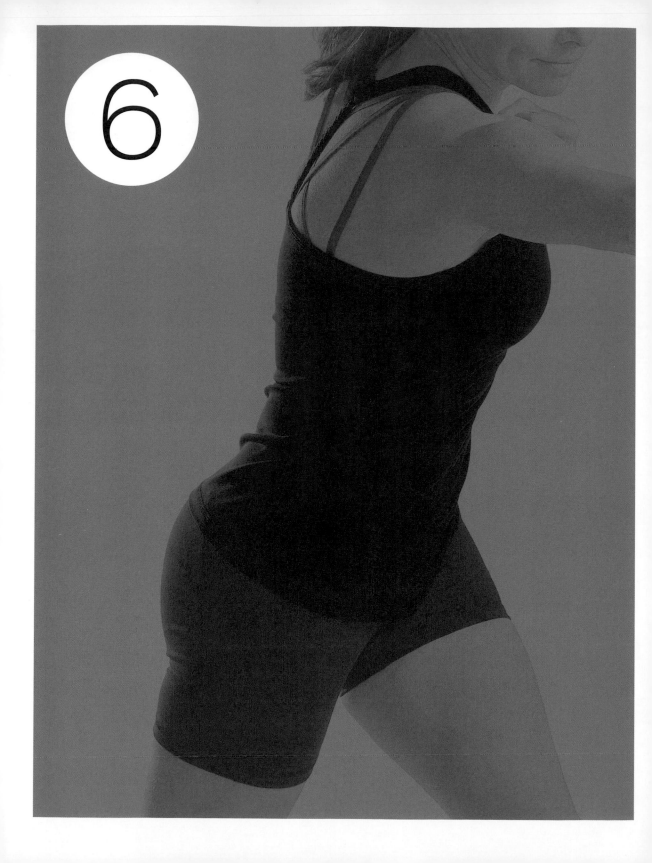

THE WORKOUTS

By this point, you've learned the theory that forms the foundation of this program, as well as the exercises and their variations. You've done the homework. Now we can have fun and finally do the workouts!

In this section you'll find several pre-set exercise routines, organized as Level 1, Level 2, and Level 3 workouts. As you move from Level 1 to Level 3, the workout gets progressively harder. But within each level, no single workout is better than another, and there is no set order that you have to follow.

Plan to spend at least two weeks on each level, doing at least three workouts per week. You may feel a little soreness afterward, but because these workouts do not stress any one body part to complete exhaustion, the soreness should resolve fairly quickly. For this reason, you could do a workout every single day, although I recommend at least one full day of rest per week.

The only guideline in choosing which workout to follow on a given day is that it should be different from the one immediately preceding it. This ensures variety in your weekly routine, which not only combats boredom but also stimulates your muscles in different ways. By varying the training stimulus in this way, you'll improve fitness and health over the long term, reduce the risk of injury, and help make this routine sustainable.

CHOOSING THE RIGHT NUMBER OF SETS AND REPS

Although the components of each workout will be a little different, some things will remain the same. Specifically, our approach to sets and repetitions will not change.

A **repetition**, or rep, is a single complete movement, from start to midpoint and back to the starting point again. A **set** is a group of repetitions performed continuously. For example, a single repetition of a push-up consists of laying facedown (start), raising up to full arm extension (midpoint), and then lowering back down again (completion). If you do this 10 times in a row, you have done one set of 10 repetitions of push-ups.

Your choice of how many repetitions and sets you do of each exercise will determine the way in which your workout will impact your body. Your goal is to

HOW CAN I MEASURE MY FITNESS?

Each workout shows a total number of sets to be performed. This "workout volume" is comprised of the number of exercises multiplied by the number of sets of each exercise. For example, a workout consisting of two sets each of ten different exercises would be expressed as 10 exercises × 2 sets, yielding a total volume of 20 sets. Along with the number of exercises, the difficulty of each exercise, number of reps, and level of resistance

when weights are used, workout volume is a measurement of fitness. As you move through the program and become more fit, workout volume increases, as does the number of exercises performed and their level of difficulty (resistance and number of reps are up to you). This progression allows each workout to build on earlier successes and prepares you to take on even more in the next one.

maximize the benefits of each repetition and each set, geting the most bang out of your workout buck.

The ideal number of sets per exercise is two. With one set, you get a tremendous improvement over doing nothing. With two sets, you're still on an improvement curve, gaining further benefit. After that, the law of diminishing returns sets in: At some point, more is not better. In fact, more can sometimes be worse. Rather than continuing to do additional sets of an exercise with no assurance that your work will yield additional benefits, you should switch to a different exercise to get a different stimulus.

That's exactly what we'll do, but not at the beginning. The first workouts start with a single set of each exercise. As you build fitness, you'll graduate to two sets per exercise. You can check your progress by noting the set totals for each workout session. (Note: Where exercises are split into left and rights sides, doing both sides counts as one set.)

Deciding how many repetitions to do in each set is trickier. The answer depends on the kind of exercise you're doing and the result you're aiming for. In traditional weightlifting, the rule of

HOW MANY REPS SHOULD I DO?

Exercises with Weights
8–12 reps with moderate
  resistance

Bodyweight Exercises
Beginner: 10–20 reps for 1 set
Advanced: 20–30 reps for 2 sets

thumb is that high resistance and low repetitions (generally between 6 and 8) help build muscle strength and size, while low resistance and high repetitions (between 12 and 20) build muscle endurance and toning. The balance between the two, where you can develop strength, endurance, *and* toning, is 8 to 12 repetitions. That's the range that you'll aim for. When a movement is difficult, or when you're trying to get acclimated to using a heavier weight, you'll be at the lower end of that range. As you improve, you'll be able to do more repetitions. When you can do more than 12 repetitions, you can increase the weight and the process begins anew. This is the essence of progressive weight-resistance training.

That solves the repetition problem for dumbbell exercises, but what about the core and balance exercises, where you'll be using your own body weight as your resistance? Since we can't increase the resistance, we'll aim to add more repetitions and take it to the upper end of our range, 20 repetitions per set. When you've achieved that goal, you can then tackle the more-advanced Level 2 and Level 3 variations. Ultimately, the goal is to be competent at the most difficult forms of each exercise for two sets of 20–30 repetitions. Then, you'll have reached the point that we were aiming for, and you can just stay at that level as you add other exercises to your routine.

Enough talk. Let's get started!

INTRODUCTORY WORKOUTS

In this series of workouts, choose the Level 1 variation of each exercise. You should be able to complete these workouts in 20 minutes or less. Despite that relatively brief amount of time, you'll be effectively challenging your body.

WORKOUT 1 (10 SETS)

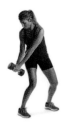

1 Push-Ups, p. 110
STRENGTH

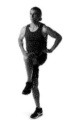

2 Side Crunches (Right), p. 124
STRENGTH

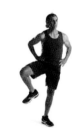

3 Supermans, p. 122 **STRENGTH**

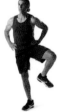

4 Side Crunches (Left), p. 124
STRENGTH

5 Standing Hurdles (Right), p. 60
BALANCE

6 Standing Hurdles (Left), p. 60 **BALANCE**

7 Reverse Hurdles (Right), p. 62
BALANCE

8 Reverse Hurdles (Left), p. 62
BALANCE

9 Dumbbell Swings (Right), p. 146 **FUNCTIONAL**

10 Dumbbell Swings (Left), p. 146 **FUNCTIONAL**

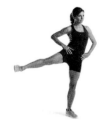

11 Side Leg Swings (Right), p. 56
BALANCE

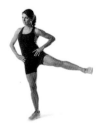

12 Side Leg Swings (Left), p. 56
BALANCE

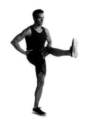

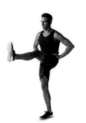

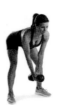

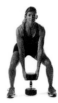

13 Front Leg Swings (Right), p. 58 **BALANCE**

14 Front Leg Swings (Left), p. 58 **BALANCE**

15 Deadlift and Front Raises, p. 144 **FUNCTIONAL**

16 Monkey Squats, p. 102 **STRENGTH**

WORKOUT 2 (11 SETS)

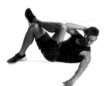

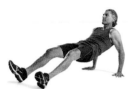

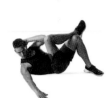

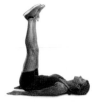

1 Crossover Crunches (Right), p. 114 **STRENGTH**

2 Hip Thrusts, p. 108 **STRENGTH**

3 Crossover Crunches (Left), p. 114 **STRENGTH**

4 Leg Raises, p. 116 **STRENGTH**

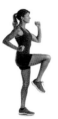

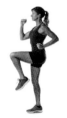

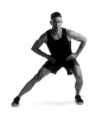

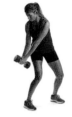

5 Step-Ups (Right), p. 142 **FUNCTIONAL**

6 Step-Ups (Left), p. 142 **FUNCTIONAL**

7 Side Lunges, p. 140 **FUNCTIONAL**

8 Dumbbell Swings (Right), p. 146 **FUNCTIONAL**

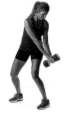

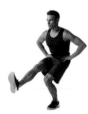

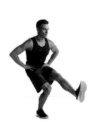

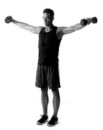

9 Dumbbell Swings (Left), p. 146 **FUNCTIONAL**

10 Pistol Squats (Right), p. 52 **BALANCE**

11 Pistol Squats (Left), p. 52 **BALANCE**

12 Lateral Raises, p. 92 **STRENGTH**

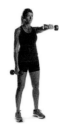 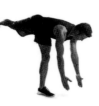 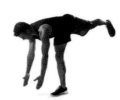 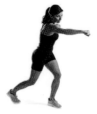

13 Front Raises, p. 94
STRENGTH

14 One-Legged
Deadlifts (Right),
p. 54 **BALANCE**

15 One-Legged
Deadlifts (Left),
p. 54 **BALANCE**

16 Dumbbell Punches
(Right), p. 152
FUNCTIONAL

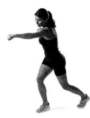

17 Dumbbell Punches
(Left), p. 152
FUNCTIONAL

WORKOUT 3 (11 SETS)

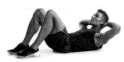

1 Crunches, p. 112
STRENGTH

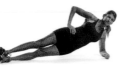

2 Side Hip Raises
(Right), p. 76
BALANCE

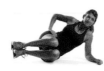

3 Side Knee Crunches
(Right), p. 86
BALANCE

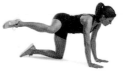

4 Fire Hydrants
(Right), p. 118
STRENGTH

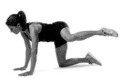

5 Fire Hydrants
(Left), p. 118
STRENGTH

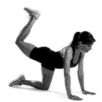

6 Donkey Kicks
(Right), p. 120
STRENGTH

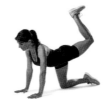

7 Donkey Kicks
(Left), p. 120
STRENGTH

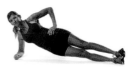

8 Side Hip Raises
(Left), p. 76 **BALANCE**

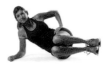

9 Side Knee Crunches
(Left), p. 86
BALANCE

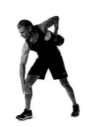

10 Lawn Mower
Rows (Right), p. 150
FUNCTIONAL

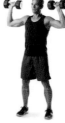

11 Lawn Mower
Rows (Left), p. 150
FUNCTIONAL

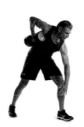

12 Standing Shoulder
Presses, p. 100
STRENGTH

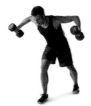

13 Low Reverse
Flyes, p. 98
STRENGTH

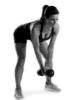

14 Deadlift and
Front Raises, p. 144
FUNCTIONAL

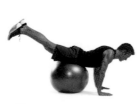

15 Reverse Leg
Raises, p. 78
BALANCE

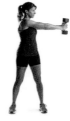

16 Torso Twists, p. 148
FUNCTIONAL

WORKOUT 4 (11 SETS)

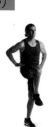

1 Lateral Raises, p. 92
STRENGTH

2 Standing Hurdles
(Right), p. 60 **BALANCE**

3 Standing Hurdles
(Left), p. 60 **BALANCE**

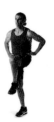

4 Front Raises, p. 94
STRENGTH

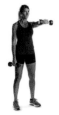

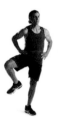

5 Reverse Hurdles
(Right), p. 62 **BALANCE**

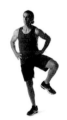

6 Reverse Hurdles
(Left), p. 62 **BALANCE**

7 High Reverse Flyes,
p. 96 **STRENGTH**

8 Side Leg Swings
(Right), p. 56 **BALANCE**

9 Side Leg Swings
(Left), p. 56 **BALANCE**

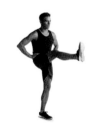

10 Low Reverse
Flyes, p. 98
STRENGTH

11 Front Leg Swings
(Right), p. 58 **BALANCE**

12 Front Leg Swings
(Left), p. 58 **BALANCE**

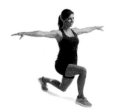

13 Walking
Lunges, p. 138
FUNCTIONAL

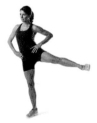

14 Deadlift and
Front Raises, p. 144
FUNCTIONAL

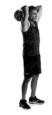

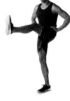

15 Triceps
Extensions, p. 90
STRENGTH

INTERMEDIATE WORKOUTS

The Level 2 series of workouts begins to raise the difficulty level, both with the number of sets and the increased complexity of each exercise. Work to perform the Level 2 variations of each exercise. You'll also perform a second set of each exercise, and we'll add some new exercises to your routine as well.

The total time that you should need of each of these workouts is approximately 20–25 minutes.

WORKOUT 1 (14 SETS)

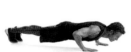 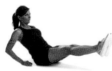 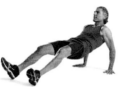 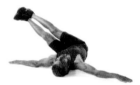

1 Push-Ups, p. 110
STRENGTH

2 Military Sit-Ups, p. 64 **BALANCE**

3 Hip Thrusts, p. 108 **STRENGTH**

4 Windshield Wipers, p. 132 **STRENGTH**

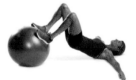 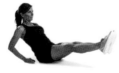 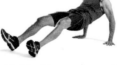 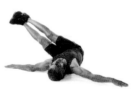

5 Stability Ball Leg Curls, p. 72 **BALANCE**

6 Military Sit-Ups, p. 64 **BALANCE**

7 Hip Thrusts, p. 108 **STRENGTH**

8 Windshield Wipers, p. 132 **STRENGTH**

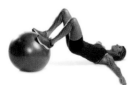 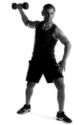 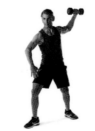 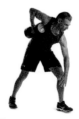

9 Stability Ball Leg Curls, p. 72 **BALANCE**

10 Discus Throws (Right), p. 154 **FUNCTIONAL**

11 Discus Throws (Left), p. 154 **FUNCTIONAL**

12 Lawn Mower Rows (Right), p. 150 **FUNCTIONAL**

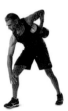

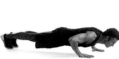

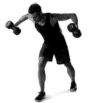

13 Lawn Mower
Rows (Left), p. 150
FUNCTIONAL

14 Push-Ups, p. 110
STRENGTH

15 High Reverse
Flyes, p. 96
STRENGTH

16 Low Reverse
Flyes, p. 98
STRENGTH

WORKOUT 2 (15 SETS)

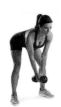

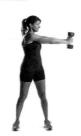

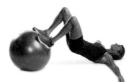

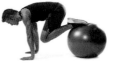

1 Deadlift and Front Raises, p. 144 **FUNCTIONAL**

2 Torso Twists, p. 148 **FUNCTIONAL**

3 Stability Ball Leg Curls, p. 72 **BALANCE**

4 Knee Tucks, p. 70 **BALANCE**

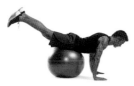

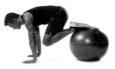

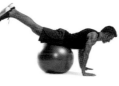

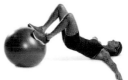

5 Reverse Leg Raises, p. 78 **BALANCE**

6 Knee Tucks, p. 70 **BALANCE**

7 Reverse Leg Raises, p. 78 **BALANCE**

8 Stability Ball Leg Curls, p. 72 **BALANCE**

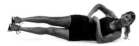

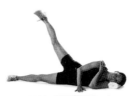

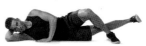

9 Side Crunches (Right), p. 124 **STRENGTH**

10 Side Hip Raises (Right), p. 76 **BALANCE**

11 Side Leg Raises (Right), p. 126 **STRENGTH**

12 Adductor Leg Raises (Right), p. 130 **STRENGTH**

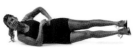

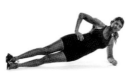

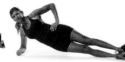

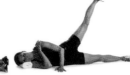

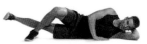

13 Side Crunches (Left), p. 124 **STRENGTH**

14 Side Hip Raises (Left), p. 76 **BALANCE**

15 Side Leg Raises (Left), p. 126 **STRENGTH**

16 Adductor Leg Raises (Left), p. 130 **STRENGTH**

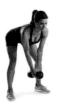

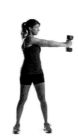

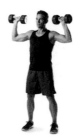

17 Deadlift and
Front Raises, p. 144
FUNCTIONAL

18 Torso Twists,
p. 148 **FUNCTIONAL**

19 Standing
Shoulder Presses
p. 100 **STRENGTH**

WORKOUT 3 (18 SETS)

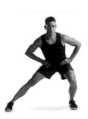

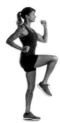

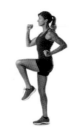

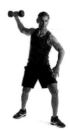

1 Side Lunges, p. 140 **FUNCTIONAL**

2 Step-Ups (Right), p. 142 **FUNCTIONAL**

3 Step-Ups (Left), p. 142 **FUNCTIONAL**

4 Discus Throws (Right), p. 154 **FUNCTIONAL**

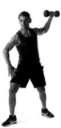

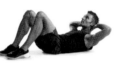

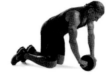

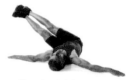

5 Discus Throws (Left), p. 154 **FUNCTIONAL**

6 Crunches, p. 112 **STRENGTH**

7 Roll Outs, p. 104 **STRENGTH**

8 Windshield Wipers, p. 132 **STRENGTH**

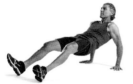

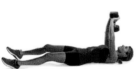

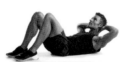

9 Hip Thrusts, p. 108 **STRENGTH**

10 Pullovers, p. 128 **STRENGTH**

11 Crunches, p. 112 **STRENGTH**

12 Roll Outs, p. 104 **STRENGTH**

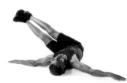

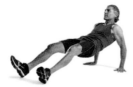

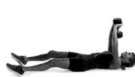

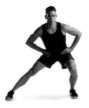

13 Windshield Wipers, p. 132 **STRENGTH**

14 Hip Thrusts, p. 108 **STRENGTH**

15 Pullovers, p. 128 **STRENGTH**

16 Side Lunges, p. 140 **FUNCTIONAL**

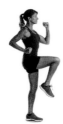 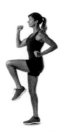 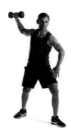 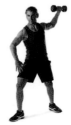

17 Step-Ups (Right), p. 142 **FUNCTIONAL**

18 Step-Ups (Left), p. 142 **FUNCTIONAL**

19 Discus Throws (Right), p. 154 **FUNCTIONAL**

20 Discus Throws (Left), p. 154 **FUNCTIONAL**

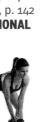 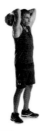

21 Deadlift and Front Raises, p. 144 **FUNCTIONAL**

22 Triceps Extensions, p. 90 **STRENGTH**

WORKOUT 4 (16 SETS)

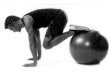

1 Knee Tucks, p. 70
BALANCE

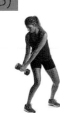

2 Dumbbell Swings
(Right), p. 146
FUNCTIONAL

3 Dumbbell Swings
(Left), p. 146
FUNCTIONAL

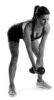

4 Deadlift and Front
Raises, p. 144
FUNCTIONAL

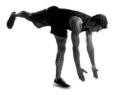

5 One-Legged
Deadlifts (Right), p. 54
BALANCE

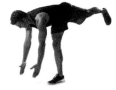

6 One-Legged
Deadlifts (Left), p. 54
BALANCE

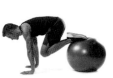

7 Knee Tucks, p. 70
BALANCE

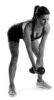

8 Standing Shoulder
Presses, p. 100
STRENGTH

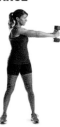

9 Torso Twists, p. 148
FUNCTIONAL

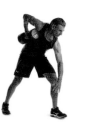

10 Lawn Mower Rows
(Right), p. 150
FUNCTIONAL

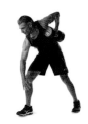

11 Lawn Mower Rows
(Left), p. 150
FUNCTIONAL

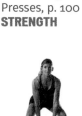

12 Monkey Squats,
p. 102 **STRENGTH**

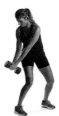

13 Dumbbell Swings
(Right), p. 146
FUNCTIONAL

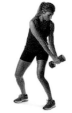

14 Dumbbell Swings
(Left), p. 146
FUNCTIONAL

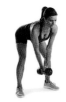

15 Deadlift and Front
Raises, p. 144
FUNCTIONAL

16 One-Legged
Deadlifts (Right),
p. 54 **BALANCE**

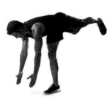

17 One-Legged Deadlifts (Left), p. 54 **BALANCE**

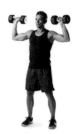

18 Standing Shoulder Presses, p. 100 **STRENGTH**

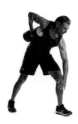

19 Torso Twists, p. 148 **FUNCTIONAL**

20 Lawn Mower Rows (Right), p. 150 **FUNCTIONAL**

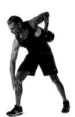

21 Lawn Mower Rows (Left), p. 150 **FUNCTIONAL**

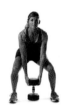

22 Monkey Squats, p. 102 **STRENGTH**

ADVANCED WORKOUTS

In this top level, you will push your limits even further. You will be doing more sets per workout, performing two sets of each exercise in more complex sequences. You'll perform additional exercises, and the workout progressions are arranged to give each muscle group less rest, which challenges them even further. You should attempt the Level 3 variation for each exercise. These workouts should take about 30–35 minutes each to perform.

WORKOUT 1 (28 SETS)

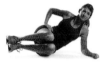 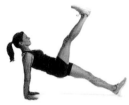 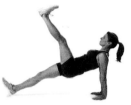

1 Side Knee Crunches (Right), p. 86 **BALANCE**

2 Hip Thrusts, p. 108 **STRENGTH**

3 Supine Plank with Leg Raises (Right), p. 74 **BALANCE**

4 Supine Plank with Leg Raises (Left), p. 74 **BALANCE**

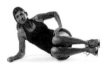 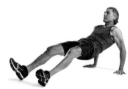 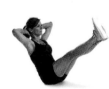 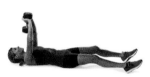

5 Side Knee Crunches (Left), p. 86 **BALANCE**

6 Hip Thrusts, p. 108 **STRENGTH**

7 V Sit-Ups, p. 80 **BALANCE**

8 Pullovers, p. 128 **STRENGTH**

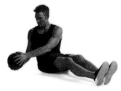 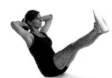 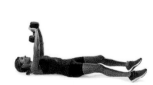 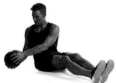

9 Russian Twists, p. 82 **BALANCE**

10 V Sit-Ups, p. 80 **BALANCE**

11 Pullovers, p. 128 **STRENGTH**

12 Russian Twists, p. 82 **BALANCE**

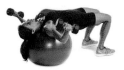 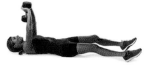 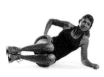 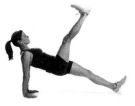

13 Dumbbell Stability Ball Flyes, p. 84 **BALANCE**

14 Pullovers, p. 128 **STRENGTH**

15 Side Knee Crunches (Right), p. 86 **BALANCE**

16 Supine Plank with Leg Raises (Right), p. 74 **BALANCE**

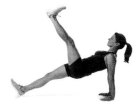 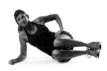 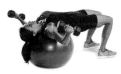

17 Supine Plank with Leg Raises (Left), p. 74 **BALANCE**

18 Side Knee Crunches (Left), p. 86 **BALANCE**

19 Dumbbell Stability Ball Flyes, p. 84 **BALANCE**

20 Lateral Raises, p. 92 **STRENGTH**

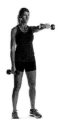 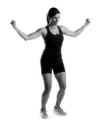 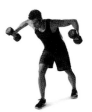 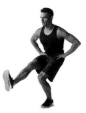

21 Front Raises, p. 94 **STRENGTH**

22 High Reverse Flyes, p. 96 **STRENGTH**

23 Low Reverse Flyes, p. 98 **STRENGTH**

24 Pistol Squats (Right), p. 52 **BALANCE**

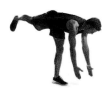 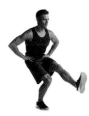 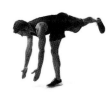 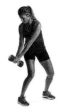

25 One-Legged Deadlifts (Right), p. 54 **BALANCE**

26 Pistol Squats (Left), p. 52 **BALANCE**

27 One-Legged Deadlifts (Left), p. 54 **BALANCE**

28 Dumbbell Swings (Right), p. 146 **FUNCTIONAL**

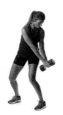

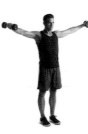

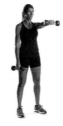

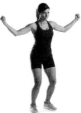

29 Dumbbell Swings (Left), p. 146 **FUNCTIONAL**

30 Lateral Raises, p. 92 **STRENGTH**

31 Front Raises, p. 94 **STRENGTH**

32 High Reverse Flyes, p. 96 **STRENGTH**

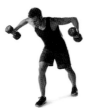

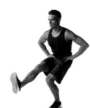

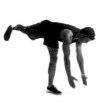

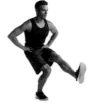

33 Low Reverse Flyes, p. 98 **STRENGTH**

34 Pistol Squats (Right), p. 52 **BALANCE**

35 One-Legged Deadlifts (Right), p. 54 **BALANCE**

36 Pistol Squats (Left), p. 52 **BALANCE**

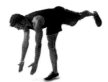

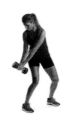

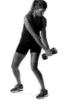

37 One-Legged Deadlifts (Left), p. 54 **BALANCE**

38 Dumbbell Swings (Right), p. 146 **FUNCTIONAL**

39 Dumbbell Swings (Left), p. 146 **FUNCTIONAL**

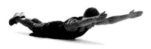

1 Roll Ups, p. 106
STRENGTH

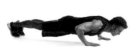

2 Push-Ups, p. 110
STRENGTH

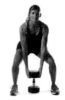

3 Monkey Squats, p. 102 **STRENGTH**

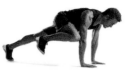

4 Mountain Climbers, p. 136
FUNCTIONAL

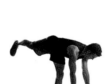

5 Supermans, p. 122
STRENGTH

6 Dumbbell Swings (Right), p. 146
FUNCTIONAL

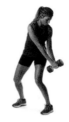

7 Dumbbell Swings (Left), p. 146
FUNCTIONAL

8 Deadlift and Front Raises, p. 144
FUNCTIONAL

9 One-Legged Deadlifts (Right), p. 54 **BALANCE**

10 One-Legged Deadlifts (Left), p. 54 **BALANCE**

11 Standing Shoulder Presses, p. 100 **STRENGTH**

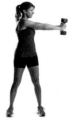

12 Torso Twists, p. 148 **FUNCTIONAL**

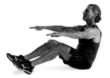

13 Roll Ups, p. 106
STRENGTH

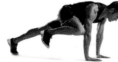

14 Push-Ups, p. 110
STRENGTH

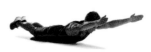

15 Mountain Climbers, p. 136
FUNCTIONAL

16 Supermans, p. 122 **STRENGTH**

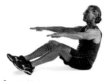
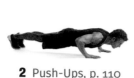

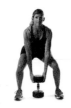 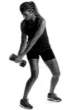 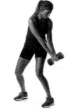 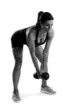

17 Monkey Squats, p. 102 **STRENGTH**

18 Dumbbell Swings (Right), p. 146 **FUNCTIONAL**

19 Dumbbell Swings (Left), p. 146 **FUNCTIONAL**

20 Deadlift and Front Raises, p. 144 **FUNCTIONAL**

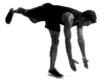 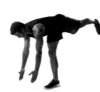 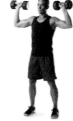 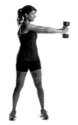

21 One-Legged Deadlifts (Right), p. 54 **BALANCE**

22 One-Legged Deadlifts (Left), p. 54 **BALANCE**

23 Standing Shoulder Presses, p. 100 **STRENGTH**

24 Torso Twists, p. 148 **FUNCTIONAL**

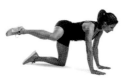 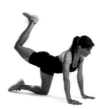 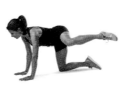 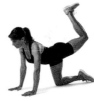

25 Fire Hydrants (Right), p. 118 **STRENGTH**

26 Donkey Kicks (Right), p. 120 **STRENGTH**

27 Fire Hydrants (Left), p. 118 **STRENGTH**

28 Donkey Kicks (Left), p. 120 **STRENGTH**

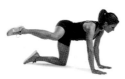 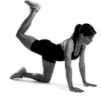 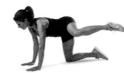 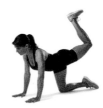

29 Fire Hydrants (Right), p. 118 **STRENGTH**

30 Donkey Kicks (Right), p. 120 **STRENGTH**

31 Fire Hydrants (Left), p. 118 **STRENGTH**

32 Donkey Kicks (Left), p. 120 **STRENGTH**

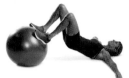

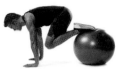

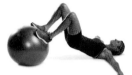

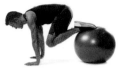

33 Stability Ball
Leg Curls, p. 72
BALANCE

34 Knee Tucks,
p. 70 **BALANCE**

35 Stability Ball
Leg Curls, p. 72
BALANCE

36 Knee Tucks,
p. 70 **BALANCE**

WORKOUT 3 (28 SETS)

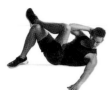 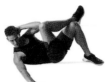 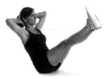 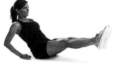

1 Crossover Crunches (Right), p. 114 **STRENGTH**

2 Crossover Crunches (Left), p. 114 **STRENGTH**

3 V Sit-Ups, p. 80 **BALANCE**

4 Military Sit-Ups, p. 64 **BALANCE**

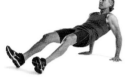 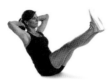 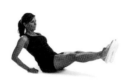 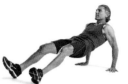

5 Hip Thrusts, p. 108 **STRENGTH**

6 V Sit-Ups, p. 80 **BALANCE**

7 Military Sit-Ups, p. 64 **BALANCE**

8 Hip Thrusts, p. 108 **STRENGTH**

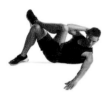 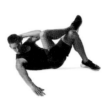 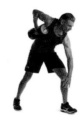 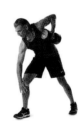

9 Crossover Crunches (Right), p. 114 **STRENGTH**

10 Crossover Crunches (Left), p. 114 **STRENGTH**

11 Lawn Mower Rows (Right), p. 150 **FUNCTIONAL**

12 Lawn Mower Rows (Left), p. 150 **FUNCTIONAL**

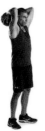 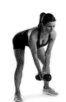 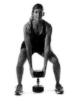 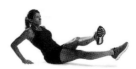

13 Triceps Extensions, p. 90 **STRENGTH**

14 Deadlift and Front Raises, p. 144 **FUNCTIONAL**

15 Monkey Squats, p. 102 **STRENGTH**

16 Leg Crossovers, p. 66 **BALANCE**

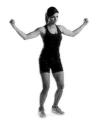

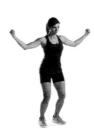

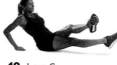

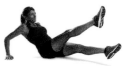

17 Flutter Kicks, p. 68
BALANCE

18 High Reverse
Flyes, p. 96
STRENGTH

19 Leg Crossovers,
p. 66 **BALANCE**

20 Flutter Kicks,
p. 68 **BALANCE**

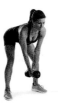

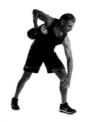

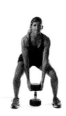

21 High Reverse
Flyes, p. 96
STRENGTH

22 Lawn Mower
Rows (Right), p. 150
FUNCTIONAL

23 Lawn Mower
Rows (Left), p. 150
FUNCTIONAL

24 Triceps
Extensions, p. 90
STRENGTH

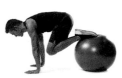

25 Deadlift and
Front Raises, p. 144
FUNCTIONAL

26 Monkey
Squats, p. 102
STRENGTH

27 Dumbbell
Stability Ball Flyes,
p. 84 **BALANCE**

28 Knee Tucks, p. 70
BALANCE

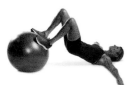

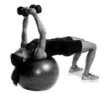

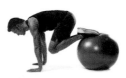

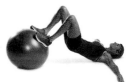

29 Stability Ball
Leg Curls, p. 72
BALANCE

30 Dumbbell
Stability Ball Flyes,
p. 84 **BALANCE**

31 Knee Tucks, p. 70
BALANCE

32 Stability Ball
Leg Curls, p. 72
BALANCE

WORKOUT 4 (28 SETS)

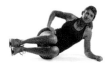

1 Side Knee Crunches (Right), p. 86 **BALANCE**

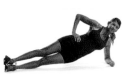

2 Side Hip Raises (Right), p. 76 **BALANCE**

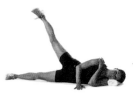

3 Side Leg Raises (Right), p. 126 **STRENGTH**

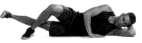

4 Adductor Leg Raises (Right), p. 130 **STRENGTH**

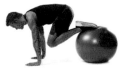

5 Knee Tucks, p. 70 **BALANCE**

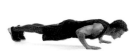

6 Push-Ups, p. 110 **STRENGTH**

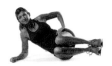

7 Side Knee Crunches (Left), p. 86 **BALANCE**

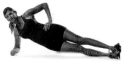

8 Side Hip Raises (Left), p. 76 **BALANCE**

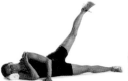

9 Side Leg Raises (Left), p. 126 **STRENGTH**

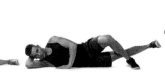

10 Adductor Leg Raises (Left), p. 130 **STRENGTH**

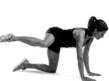

11 Fire Hydrants (Right), p. 118 **STRENGTH**

12 Donkey Kicks (Right), p. 120 **STRENGTH**

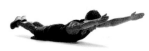

13 Supermans, p. 122 **STRENGTH**

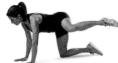

14 Fire Hydrants (Left), p. 118 **STRENGTH**

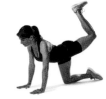

15 Donkey Kicks (Left), p. 120 **STRENGTH**

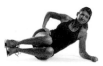

16 Side Knee Crunches (Right), p. 86 **BALANCE**

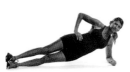

17 Side Hip Raises (Right), p. 76 **BALANCE**

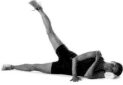

18 Side Leg Raises (Right), p. 126 **STRENGTH**

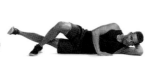

19 Adductor Leg Raises (Right), p. 130 **STRENGTH**

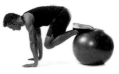

20 Knee Tucks, p. 70 **BALANCE**

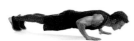

21 Push-Ups, p. 110 **STRENGTH**

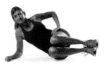

22 Side Knee Crunches (Left), p. 86 **BALANCE**

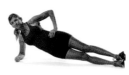

23 Side Hip Raises (Left), p. 76 **BALANCE**

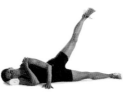

24 Side Leg Raises (Left), p. 126 **STRENGTH**

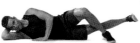

25 Adductor Leg Raises (Left), p. 130 **STRENGTH**

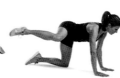

26 Fire Hydrants (Right), p. 118 **STRENGTH**

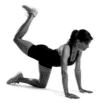

27 Donkey Kicks (Right), p. 120 **STRENGTH**

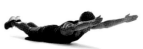

28 Supermans, p. 122 **STRENGTH**

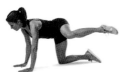

29 Fire Hydrants (Left), p. 118 **STRENGTH**

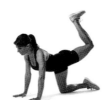

30 Donkey Kicks (Left), p. 120 **STRENGTH**

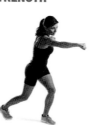

31 Dumbbell Punches (Right), p. 152 **FUNCTIONAL**

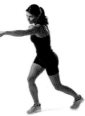

32 Dumbbell Punches (Left), p. 152 **FUNCTIONAL**

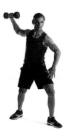
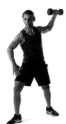
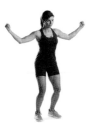
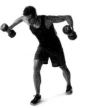

33 Discus Throws (Right), p. 154 **FUNCTIONAL**

34 Discus Throws (Left), p. 154 **FUNCTIONAL**

35 High Reverse Flyes, p. 96 **STRENGTH**

36 Low Reverse Flyes, p. 98 **STRENGTH**

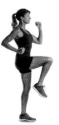
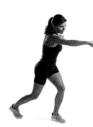
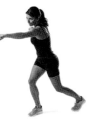

37 Step-Ups (Right), p. 142 **FUNCTIONAL**

38 Step-Ups (Left), p. 142 **FUNCTIONAL**

39 Dumbbell Punches (Right), p. 152 **FUNCTIONAL**

40 Dumbbell Punches (Left), p. 152 **FUNCTIONAL**

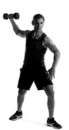
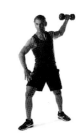
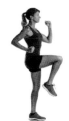
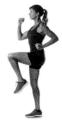

41 Discus Throws (Right), p. 154 **FUNCTIONAL**

42 Discus Throws (Left), p. 154 **FUNCTIONAL**

43 Step-Ups (Right), p. 142 **FUNCTIONAL**

44 Step-Ups (Left), p. 142 **FUNCTIONAL**

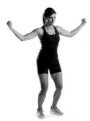
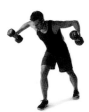

45 High Reverse Flyes, p. 96 **STRENGTH**

46 Low Reverse Flyes, p. 98 **STRENGTH**

WHEN NOT TO WORK OUT

For many of us, the toughest part about maintaining an exercise routine is finding the time and motivation to stick with it. Family commitments, work deadlines, and social obligations sometimes seem to conspire against our best intentions, leaving us feeling guilty and defeated when we fail to do the workout we promised ourselves we would not miss.

Sometimes, however, we encounter the opposite problem. We find ourselves ready and willing to hit our exercise routine, but the wisest course of action would be to skip the workout. Here are some situations when appropriate discretion requires you to skip your scheduled training session.

Injury. Soreness is a common result of exercise, and it's to be expected. When we challenge a muscle by working it beyond its capacity, we create micro-tears in the muscle fibers. During the healing process, the body resculpts that muscle to increase its capacity to perform work and meet this challenge in the future. The nature of that change depends on the particular training stimulus. So, for example, a workout that emphasizes cardio exercise will result in improved endurance, while a routine that emphasizes weightlifting will result in muscle cells that are slightly bigger and slightly stronger.

Soreness that results from these workouts should be general achiness throughout the targeted muscle group. After a full day's rest, it should feel better. Although it might seem counterintuitive, working a sore muscle group again at that point actually helps. That's because the muscle fibers may have formed adhesions to one another as they healed, causing them to stick together like overcooked spaghetti. This can reduce the range of motion in the related joint and cause discomfort. Exercise breaks up those adhesions and helps restore proper range of motion. (Incidentally, deep tissue massage does the same thing, which is why you might feel uncomfortable, and even in pain, during the session but much better afterward.)

An injured muscle, however, feels entirely different. Instead of experiencing general soreness, you feel a sharp pain in a specific location. Also, although a day off from exercise often alleviates run-of-the-mill soreness, an injury probably won't get better after just a day's rest. Instead, it will continue to hurt. Working it further at this point will only further damage the muscle tissue. The better course of treatment is to take more time off and to seek medical attention if it doesn't improve after several days.

Illness. Here's a good rule of thumb when it comes to illness: If you've simply got congestion and a stuffy or running nose, go ahead and do your scheduled workout. Exercise won't make things worse, and the increased oxygen intake from exercise might actually make you feel better.

If, however, you've got a scratchy or sore throat, or are running a fever with aches and pains, take a day off from all exercise. Exercise temporarily suppresses your immune system (although it improves your immune function over the long term), and since your immune system is already taxed from fighting an infection, your exercise session will only make it that much harder for your body to recover and get well. Instead of working out, rest up and get healthy.

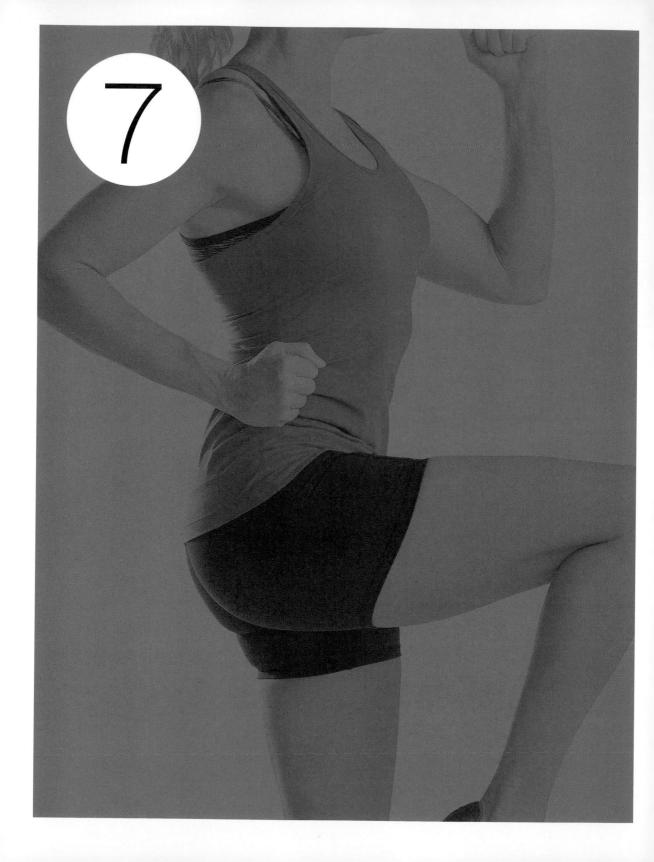

STRENGTH
FOR THE LONG TERM

By the time you read this chapter, you may well have progressed through the Level 3 workouts listed in Chapter 6. If so, congratulations! So what's your next move? You have several options:

- Continue rotating through the Level 3 workouts, adding variety by choosing different variations of each exercise for each session.
- Combine the Level 1 workouts into one challenging routine and add that into your workout list.
- Combine two Level 2 workouts to further expand your list of workout choices.

Any of these options will keep you on the path to building and maintaining strength. But there's another option available to you as well: designing your own training sessions. By following the simple guidelines in this chapter, you can create hundreds of effective workouts.

COLOR YOUR WORKOUT

As discussed in Chapter 4, a balanced workout should be a combination of functionality, strength, and balance exercises in order to develop a broad fitness base. That chapter introduced our color-coding system, which was used in Chapter 5 to designate each exercise's primary characteristic.

Now it's time to put this system to work for you. In order to design a workout that challenges and improves all of the target areas—strength, balance, and functionality—you simply need to choose exercises from each of these color-coded categories.

Just as with the preset workouts in Chapter 6, the aim is to include at least two exercises from each color. Since many of the exercises in this book fall in the strength category, those will likely make up the lion's share of each of your workouts. But by also including functional and balance exercises, you ensure that you are working toward meeting all of your strength training goals with every workout.

MIX IT UP

To maintain interest and variety, aim to avoid doing the same workout twice in a row. With 50 exercises to choose from, the possible combinations of exercises are nearly endless. But mixing things up isn't just about keeping you from getting bored. It's about continuously giving your body new challenges, which keeps it from getting complacent. As far as your body is concerned, change is a good thing. Keep your body guessing, and it will continue to deliver results.

You might think that incorporating constant change into your routine would be mentally exhausting, but actually the opposite is true. It doesn't take much variety from workout to workout to keep things feeling fresh; sometimes adding or deleting just a few exercises can make all the difference.

Here are some additional ideas that you can try to spice things up.

Change the number of repetitions. The sweet spot when using weights, between encouraging strength gains on the one hand and improving muscle tone and endurance on the other hand, is found between 8 and 12 repetitions per set. Occasionally, though—no more than about once per month—you should go outside that range, especially when using dumbbells, just to shake things up. For example, use heavier dumbbells and perform 4–6 repetitions per set. Or choose lighter resistance and do 20 repetitions in every set.

Change the number of sets. The goal we set earlier for ourselves was around 20 total sets per workout, comprised of two sets per exercise. Just as with the number of repetitions that you perform, this goal is subject to change as well. You can raise the total to 30 sets or more, or drop it down to just 10–12 hard sets.

Another alternative would be to do only one set of any exercise, but to add more exercises. A subtle benefit from this format is to remove the natural (but often unrecognized) tendency to hold back when you're doing multiple sets as you pace yourself for the second set. Removing the second set frees you to push harder, since you'll know that you won't have to return to that exercise during that workout.

Change the level of difficulty. The idea behind working through the routines in Chapter 6 is to progress from Level 1 to Level 2 and Level 3 with each exercise. However, you should continue to think of all three forms as viable options from which you can choose in order to mod-ulate the difficulty of your workout, as well as to maintain variety. For example, try using Level 1 forms as a warm-up, and then switch to Level 2 or 3 for a second set of each exercise. Or alternate between easier and harder versions of an exercise during the workout.

Finally, try doing the Level 3 version of one group of exercises—say, the balance work—but do the Level 1 or 2 forms for all other exercises scheduled for that session. This moderates the difficulty of the workout by alternating harder challenges with easier challenges, and provides you with productive recovery time between hard sets. Similarly, you can alternate complex exercises with simple single-joint exercises.

CLUSTER EXERCISES

You might have noticed that the preset workouts group similar exercises together. This is not a coincidence. I call this "clustering," and I use it to decrease unproductive time between sets and thereby increase the intensity of the workout.

Clustering works by combining certain exercises into mini-workouts, or circuits. These circuits are designed to reduce the movement needed to get from one exercise to another. For example, if you were to perform a Russian twist and then a dumbbell pullover with a leg raise, you could move from one set to the next with no break in between. But if you were to add in a one-legged deadlift between the two, you would have to stand up, get into position for the deadlift, and then return to your exercise mat after the deadlifts are completed.

Although it's true that you would be getting some training benefit from simply getting up and sitting down again, that movement wouldn't be as effective or precise as performing one of our listed exercises. The net effect of getting up and sitting down is that it lengthens the amount of time that it takes to do the workout and also gives you a breather right in the middle of it. If you need a short breather, that's fine. But if not, then you are just wasting time during the workout and letting your body rest when it should be getting a training stimulus instead.

As you design your own workouts, consider clustering exercises in this manner:

- Floor exercises, with dumbbell floor exercises as one subset and body-weight core exercises as another

- Standing balance work
- Standing dumbbell work
- Simple single-joint movements

Regarding difficulty, bear in mind this guiding principle: The point of your workouts is to attain the right level of effort. If you push your body correctly, it responds by improving. Push too hard, however, and you risk injury. It's important to recognize when you need to slow things down a bit so that you don't give your body more than it can handle.

If needed, you can design your workout to allow for a quick rest between hard efforts by stacking particular exercises together. For example, if you performed Russian twists and pullovers with leg raises back-to-back, as described above, you could then do a standing balance exercise, using the time spent standing up as an opportunity to catch your breath before the next big effort.

ALTERNATING BODY PARTS

Performing similar exercises consecutively is one way to increase your workout challenge. Doing the exact opposite can also raise the intensity of your workout. By targeting different body parts from set to set, you allow one group of muscles to rest while working another. The net effect is to maintain nearly constant motion, which reduces wasted time, keeps your heart rate elevated throughout the workout, and makes your workout more effective and efficient.

Here's an example of how this might work: Do one set of push-ups to work your push muscles (chest, front shoulders, and triceps), and follow immediately with one set of lawn mower rows to work your pull muscles (back and biceps). Although this routine requires you to stand up between sets, you are challenging two very different muscle groups back-to-back, allowing you the opportunity to work each of them harder that you might otherwise be able to do.

Whatever options you choose to build and vary your workouts, it all boils down to this: When you organize your workout routine, make sure to see not just the trees but also the forest. A good workout has a flow, just like a piece of classical music. One exercise should lead naturally into the next, husbanding your energy expenditure so you get the most out of your performance.

Remember, as long as you're performing the exercises correctly and using good form, there is really no bad routine. There are only those that you'll find more effective and enjoyable, and those that you'll find to be less so. Keep a sense of adventure; experiment and have fun.

JACK LALANNE

When I was growing up in the 1970s, I would occasionally come across a show on TV featuring a man in a light-colored jumpsuit showing viewers (presumably bored housewives, as this was a midday, midweek program) how to exercise. I looked at him as I would look at an old vaudevillian, not sure why it was funny, but sure that it wasn't to be taken seriously.

I could not have been more wrong. As I found out many years later, Jack LaLanne was an innovator in the fitness industry and a lifelong advocate and practitioner for a healthy, active, and adventurous lifestyle. In a time before Nike, he just did it. He was the real deal.

Born in 1914 in San Francisco of French immigrants, Jack was a self-described sugarholic as a teenager, with behavioral issues that led to violence that he directed at others and himself. At 15, he heard a lecture by a noted nutritionist that changed his life. He dedicated himself to eating fresh, whole foods, and he discovered weight lifting and exercising. He was transformed. He returned to high school and made the football team, and then went to college and became a doctor of chiropractic medicine.

At 21, he opened the nation's first fitness gym, in Oakland, California, and followed that up with dozens more. Not content with the equipment then available, he designed his own machines and pulley systems, which he refused to patent because he wanted others to build them as well. He became a vocal advocate for an active, healthy lifestyle, preaching that everyone—women as well as men—should lift weights and exercise.

LaLanne's views were not widely shared at the time. Doctors rejected his advice and instructed their patients to avoid his gyms. They said that if people followed LaLanne's programs, they would risk having a heart attack and decreased libido. LaLanne rejected these criticisms. Instead, he doubled down, refusing to eat processed foods and marketing his own juicer. He expanded his chain of gyms, eventually selling them to a company that became Bally Total Fitness.

In 1953, LaLanne created his iconic television show, paying out of his own pocket for a 15-minute morning time slot. In 1959, the ABC network picked up the show. It aired for another 28 years, becoming TV's longest-running exercise show.

Eventually, the rest of the country caught up with LaLanne, and he became a household name associated with health and strength. He was recognized with a long list of awards and honors, including, at age 88, a star on the Hollywood Walk of Fame, which he inaugurated with a set of push-ups at his induction ceremony.

LaLanne's approach to life was to treat it like it was an athletic event. "You've got to exercise," he said. "Your health account is like a bank account. The more you put in, the more you can take out."

Among his many achievements was a tradition of performing public feats of strength well into his later years. These included:

- Setting a world record by swimming the length of the Golden Gate Bridge with 140 pounds of air tanks strapped to his back
- Swimming from Alcatraz Island to Fisherman's Wharf in San Francisco while handcuffed
- Performing 1,033 push-ups in 23 minutes on live TV
- Swimming the Golden Gate strait while towing a 2,500-pound cabin cruiser a total of 6.5 miles after currents threw him off course
- Performing 1,000 jumping jacks and 1,000 pull-ups in one hour
- Towing 10 boats in North Miami, Florida, pulling a total of 77 people
- At age 70, towing 70 rowboats on a 1-mile swim from Long Beach Harbor, California, to the moored liner *Queen Mary*

LaLanne once said, "I'd hate to die; it would ruin my image." Nevertheless, he passed away in 2011, at age 96, from respiratory failure due to pneumonia. He had been sick for a week but had refused to see a doctor. Reportedly, he had performed his exercise routine the day before his death.

LaLanne's life stands as a tribute to health, but he didn't work out just for the sake of working out. Instead, he used exercise as a springboard into a world of adventures and challenges. Undeterred by both critics and age itself, he remained active and vital into his 10th decade. He had ageless strength before the concept was even invented.

ACKNOWLEDGMENTS

The inspiration for this book came from my clients, several of whom are in their 60s and 70s. They are as different from each other as they can be, but what they all have in common is a love of life. They work out not just to look good in the gym, but so they can do fun things outside the gym.

From them I've learned that the challenge isn't just to build and maintain functional strength, increase bone density, or improve balance. It's to use improvements in these areas to work toward a far more important goal: to live a meaningful, productive, and adventurous life.

This doesn't happen by accident. To paraphrase the famous football coach Vince Lombardi, adventure is where preparation meets opportunity. When your body is strong and fit, you can take on any challenge that captures your imagination.

Having worked with a large number of athletes of all abilities and ages, I've learned that achievement is rooted in a simple formula. To succeed at anything, including fitness, you need two things: greed for improvement and an appreciation for what you've already accomplished.

Greed motivates us to work hard to reach our goals. Without greed for more adventure, we lack the drive necessary to get there. If all we have is greed, however, we'll never be satisfied, so we also need to appreciate the gains we've made. But if all we have is satisfaction, we become complacent.

The key is to have greed and appreciation in equal proportions. Only then can we be happy with what we've achieved while remaining eager to achieve even more.

This is the goal that my clients have inspired in me. It is to them that I dedicate this book.

I also owe a great debt to my wife and partner, Stephanie. People say that a spouse is someone who knows you really well but who loves you anyway. With Stephanie, I hit the jackpot!

I'm also thankful for the whole team at VeloPress, but especially to Casey Blaine, who truly gets it, lives it, and shares it.

Don't live to exercise; exercise to live, truly and fully. Now take what you've learned in this book and go do something!

EXERCISE INDEX

EXERCISE	PAGE	PURPOSE	EQUIPMENT NEEDED		
			LEVEL 1	LEVEL 2	LEVEL 3
Adductor Leg Raises	130	STRENGTH		Dumbbell	Dumbbell
Crossover Crunches	114	STRENGTH			BOSU
Crunches	112	STRENGTH			Stability ball
Deadlift and Front Raises	144	FUNCTIONAL	Dumbbell	Dumbbell	BOSU
Discus Throws	154	FUNCTIONAL		Dumbbell	Dumbbell
Donkey Kicks	120	STRENGTH		BOSU	BOSU
Dumbbell Punches	152	FUNCTIONAL		Dumbbell	Dumbbell
Dumbbell Stability Ball Flyes	84	BALANCE		Dumbbell	BOSU
Dumbbell Swings	146	FUNCTIONAL	Dumbbell	Dumbbell, stability ball	BOSU
Fire Hydrants	118	STRENGTH		BOSU	BOSU
Flutter Kicks	68	BALANCE			Dumbbell
Front Leg Swings	58	BALANCE			BOSU
Front Raises	94	STRENGTH	Dumbbell	Dumbbell	Dumbbell, BOSU

Continues

Continued

EXERCISE	PAGE	PURPOSE	EQUIPMENT NEEDED		
			LEVEL 1	LEVEL 2	LEVEL 3
High Reverse Flyes	96	STRENGTH		Dumbbell	Dumbbell, BOSU
Hip Thrusts	108	STRENGTH			BOSU
Knee Tucks	70	BALANCE	Stability ball	Stability ball	Stability ball, BOSU
Lateral Raises	92	STRENGTH	Dumbbell	Dumbbell	Dumbbell, BOSU
Lawn Mower Rows	150	FUNCTIONAL	Dumbbell	Dumbbell	Dumbbell
Leg Crossovers	66	BALANCE			Dumbbell
Leg Raises	116	STRENGTH		Stability ball	
Low Reverse Flyes	98	STRENGTH	Dumbbell	Dumbbell	Dumbbell, BOSU
Military Sit-Ups	64	BALANCE			Dumbbell
Monkey Squats	102	STRENGTH		Dumbbell	Dumbbell, BOSU
Mountain Climbers	136	FUNCTIONAL			
One-Legged Deadlifts	54	BALANCE		Dumbbell or medicine ball	Dumbbell or medicine ball, BOSU
Pistol Squats	52	BALANCE		Dumbbell or medicine ball	Dumbbell or medicine ball, BOSU
Pullovers	128	STRENGTH	Dumbbell	Dumbbell	Dumbbell, BOSU

EXERCISE	PAGE	PURPOSE	EQUIPMENT NEEDED		
			LEVEL 1	LEVEL 2	LEVEL 3
Push-Ups	110	STRENGTH			
Reverse Hurdles	62	BALANCE			BOSU
Reverse Leg Raises	78	BALANCE	Stability ball	Stability ball	Stability ball, BOSU
Roll Outs	104	STRENGTH	Ab wheel	Ab wheel	Ab wheel
Roll Ups	106	STRENGTH			
Russian Twists	82	BALANCE	Dumbbell or medicine ball	Dumbbell or medicine ball	Dumbbell or medicine ball
Side Crunches	124	STRENGTH			BOSU
Side Hip Raises	76	BALANCE			BOSU
Side Knee Crunches	86	BALANCE		BOSU	BOSU
Side Leg Raises	126	STRENGTH			
Side Leg Swings	56	BALANCE			BOSU
Side Lunges	140	FUNCTIONAL			Dumbbell or medicine ball
Stability Ball Leg Curls	72	BALANCE	Stability ball	Stability ball	Stability ball, BOSU
Standing Hurdles	60	BALANCE			BOSU

Continues

Continued

EXERCISE	PAGE	PURPOSE	EQUIPMENT NEEDED		
			LEVEL 1	LEVEL 2	LEVEL 3
Standing Shoulder Presses	100	STRENGTH	Dumbbell	Dumbbell	Dumbbell
Step-Ups	142	FUNCTIONAL			
Supermans	122	STRENGTH		BOSU	Dumbbell, BOSU
Supine Plank with Leg Raises	74	BALANCE			BOSU
Torso Twists	148	FUNCTIONAL	Dumbbell	Dumbbell	Dumbbell
Triceps Extensions	90	STRENGTH	Dumbbell or medicine ball	Dumbbell or medicine ball	Dumbbell or medicine ball, BOSU
V Sit-Ups	80	BALANCE			
Walking Lunges	138	FUNCTIONAL		Dumbbell	Dumbbell
Windshield Wipers	132	STRENGTH			Stability ball

NOTES

INTRODUCTION: AGING BODIES, AGELESS STRENGTH

1. See John E. Morley et al., "Potentially Predictive and Manipulable Blood Serum Correlates of Aging in the Healthy Human Male: Progressive Decreases in Bioavailable Testosterone, Dehydroepiandrosterone Sulfate, and the Ratio of Insulin-Like Growth Factor 1 to Growth Hormone," *Proceedings of the National Academy of Sciences of the United States of America* 94, no. 14: 7537–7754.

2. For a very interesting and fun discussion on the effects of weightlessness, see Chris Hadfield, *An Astronaut's Guide to Life on Earth* (Boston: Little, Brown, 2013).

3. See Kirsten Weir, "The Exercise Effect," *American Psychological Association Monitor on Psychology* 42, no. 11 (December 2011).

4. Physical peak ranges from age 23 to 28. See, for example, Stephen C. Hollings, Will G. Hopkins, and Patria A. Hume, "Age at Peak Performance of Successful Track and Field Athletes," *International Journal of Sports Science and Coaching* 9 no. 4 (September 2014): 651–661.

CHAPTER 1: A NEW WAY OF UNDERSTANDING EXERCISE

1. "Aging is associated with progressive losses in function across multiple systems, including sensation, cognition, memory, [and] motor control. . . . [A] new viewpoint—based upon decades of research in neuroscience, experimental psychology, and other related fields—argues that as people age . . . [f]our core factors—reduced schedules of brain activity, noisy processing, weakened neuromodulatory control, and negative learning—interact to create a self-reinforcing downward spiral of degraded brain function in older adults. . . . Studies of adult brain plasticity have shown that substantial improvement in function and/or recovery from losses in sensation, cognition, memory, motor control, and affect should be possible, using appropriately designed behavioral training paradigms." Merzenich Mahncke Bronstone, "Brain Plasticity and Functional Losses in the Aged: Scientific Bases for a Novel Intervention," *Progress in Brain Research* 157 (2006): 81–109; emphasis added.

CHAPTER 2: CHANGES AND CHALLENGES

1. B. Newman, L. Haggerty, B. Goodpaster, T. Harris, S. Kritchevsky, M. Nevitt, T. P. Miles, and M. Visser, "Strength and Muscle Quality in a Well-Functioning Cohort of Older Adults: The Health, Aging and Body Composition Study," *Journal of the American Geriatrics Society* (March 2003).

2. A. P. Wroblewski, F. Amati, M. A. Smiley, B. Goodpaster, and V. Wright, "Chronic Exercise Preserves Lean Muscle Mass in Masters Athletes," *The Physician and Sports Medicine* 39, no. 3 (September 2011): 172–178.

3. See the recommendations of the American College of Sports Medicine (http://www.acsm.org), the American Heart Association (https://www.heart.org/HEARTORG/HealthyLiving/PhysicalActivity/FitnessBasics/Fitness-Basics_UCM_462340_SubHomePage.jsp), and the U.S. Department of Health and Human Services (https://health.gov/paguidelines).

4. S. Going, T. Lohman, L. Houtkooper et al., "Effects of Exercise on Bone Mineral Density in Calcium-Replete Postmenopausal Women with and without Hormone Replacement Therapy," *Osteoporosis International* 14 (2003): 637; R. E. Rikli and B. G. McManis, "Effects of Exercise on Bone Mineral Content in Postmenopausal Women," *Research Quarterly for Exercise and Sport* 61, no. 3: 243–249 (1990).

5. Douglas Paddon-Jones, Kevin R. Short, Wayne W. Campbell, Elena Volpi, and Robert R. Wolfe, "Role of Dietary Protein in the Sarcopenia of Aging," *The American Journal of Clinical Nutrition* 87, no. 5 (May 2008): 1562S–1566S.

6. Judith A. Beto, "The Role of Calcium in Human Aging," *Clinical Nutrition Research* 4, no. 1 (January 2015): 1–8.

7. Center for Disease Control, "Important Facts about Falls," http://www.cdc.gov/homeandrecreationalsafety/falls/adultfalls.html.

8. B. G. Vopat, S. A. Klinge, P. K. McClure, and P. D. Fadale, "The Effects of Fitness on the Aging Process," *Journal of the American Academy of Orthopaedic Surgeons* 22, no. 9 (September 2014): 576–585.

9. P. A. Beere, S. D. Russell, M. C. Morey, D. W. Kitzman, and M. B. Higginbotham, "Aerobic Exercise Training Can Reverse Age-Related Peripheral Circulatory Changes in Healthy Older Men," *Circulation* 100, no. 10 (1999): 1085–1094.

10. American College of Sports Medicine, "ACSM Issues New Recommendations on Quantity and Quality of Exercise," http://www.acsm.org/about-acsm/media-room/news-releases/2011/08/01/acsm-issues-new-recommendations-on-quantity-and-quality-of-exercise.

ABOUT THE AUTHOR

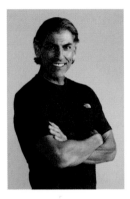

Jeff Horowitz is an author, editor, speaker, and youth development program director with over 20 years' experience in the fitness industry. Formerly a practicing attorney, Jeff quit law to share his passion for endurance sport and healthy living. He's now a certified triathlon, running, and cycling coach, as well as a personal trainer.

Jeff's books include *Quick Strength for Runners*, *Smart Marathon Training: Run Your Best Without Running Yourself Ragged*, and *My First 100 Marathons: 2,620 Miles with an Obsessive Runner*.

Jeff has run more than 180 marathons, completing at least one marathon in every state and on six continents, including Antarctica. He has also competed in ultramarathons, stage races in the Himalayas and through the Rockies, and long-distance cycling events. He lives in Washington, D.C., with his wife, the artist and teacher Stephanie Kay, and their 11-year-old son, Alex.

Visit Jeff and read his blog at www.RunHorowitz.com.